THE PRIMAL GOURMET COOKBOOK

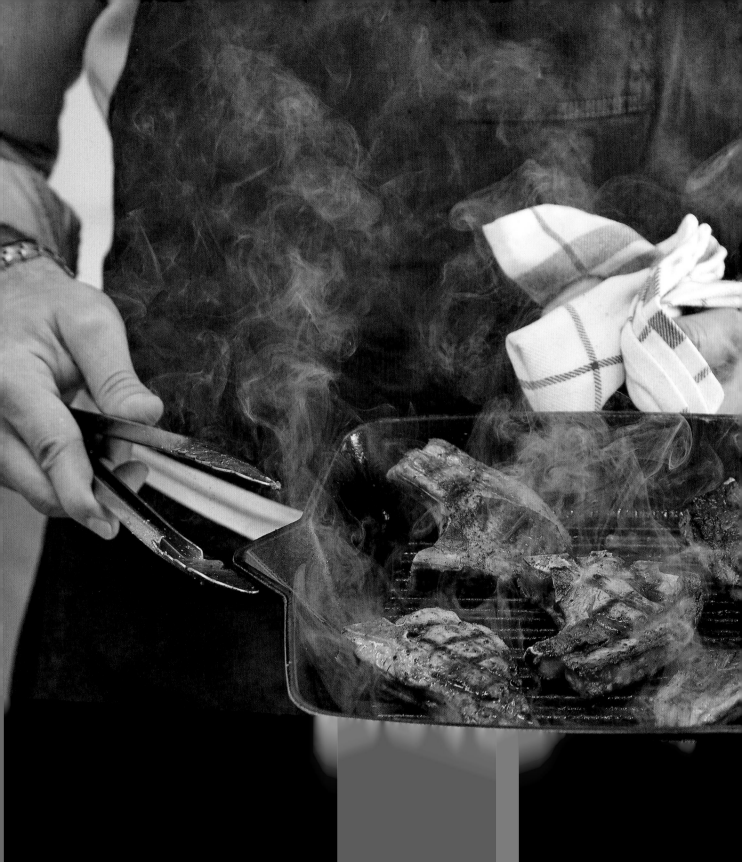

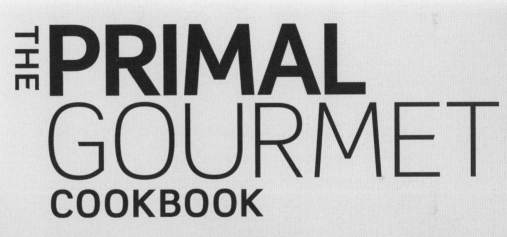

THE PRIMAL GOURMET
COOKBOOK

It's Not a Diet if It's Delicious

RONNY JOSEPH LVOVSKI

Photography by Donna Griffith

HOUGHTON MIFFLIN HARCOURT

BOSTON NEW YORK 2020

For information about permissions to reproduce selections
from this book, write to trade.premissions@hmhco.com or to
Permissions, Houghton Mifflin Harcourt Publishing Company,
3 Park Avenue, 19th Floor, New York, New York 10016.

hmhbooks.com

Library of Congress Cataloguing-in-Publication Data is available.

ISBN 978-0-358-16027-4 (POB)

ISBN 978-0-358-16030-4 (ebook)

Book design by Jennifer K. Beal Davis

Printed in China

TLF 10 9 8 7 6 5 4 3 2 1

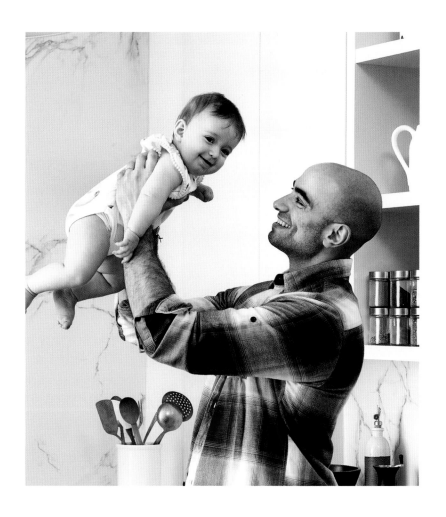

To my daughter, Sofia.
Work hard, be kind, and
never take no for an answer.

CONTENTS

SAUCES, DRESSINGS, AND SPICE BLENDS || 229

FOREWORD

If you've done the Whole30 or just love our recipes, you've certainly seen Ronny during one of his famous Whole30 Recipes Instagram takeovers. He's always the most popular host of the year, garnering hundreds of enthusiastic comments and new followers. Every time he appears, I get at least a dozen messages from his legion of fans: "This man needs his own cookbook." It's taken everything I have over the last year not to reply back, "Yeah, we're WAY ahead of you."

It's quite possible, however, that I'm at the top of the Ronny Joseph Lvovski Fan Club. Every time I see his smiling face on social media, hear his Latin-inspired kitchen music, or watch him take a huge bite out of a freshly made dish, I beam along with him. Ronny is the kind of home chef who inspires pure joy in the kitchen, with his love of fresh ingredients, his encouragement to try new things, and the way he unabashedly savors the heck out of his own finished product. Honestly, if his recipes were just pretty good, I'd still be cooking along with him, he's that charming and engaging. But his recipes are SO MUCH MORE than just pretty good.

As you flip through this book, you'll immediately see what I mean. Meals are a riot of textures and colors, flavors are thrown together in casual but creative ways, and classics are reinvented with modern twists and zesty accents.

Look deeper, though, and you'll find a steadfast commitment to virtuosity in all of Ronny's cooking techniques. Just follow his instructions and, magically, steaks are perfectly seared, veggies are crisp-tender, and even hard-boiled eggs have the perfect jammy center. The end result is that his meals taste even better than they look on these pages.

Now, onto the good stuff. Every time I launch a new Whole30 Endorsed cookbook, you ask me, "What are your favorite recipes?" and I always sigh with the impossibility of the task. It's so hard to narrow it down, but I'll give you a few standouts from Ronny's book.

First, the Grilled Shrimp Cobb (page 12) is one of those fancy-looking dishes that is surprisingly fast to pull together, and it makes for a hearty brunch dish. The spicy + sweet combo of the Mojo Loco Chicken Wings (page 46) is heaven in the oven, spoken as someone who is a recent convert to all things jalapeño. The Picadillo (page 96) is my son's most-requested dish, especially with pan-fried plantains on the side. (Olives and raisins together --who knew?) And we spatchcocked a chicken using the technique on page 64 for Thanksgiving this year, mostly just to keep saying the word *spatchcock*, but also because Ronny's surprisingly easy technique gave us insanely crispy skin and tender, moist meat.

I could fill the rest of this page with recipes you should make, but I guarantee you're ready to turn the page and dive in. As you do, allow yourself to receive the energy, vibrancy, and joy spilling out of these pages. This isn't just a cookbook; it's a journey into the way cooking at home should be --with a dash of spice, a splash of oil, a quick little salsa step, and a huge grin on your face.

Best in health,

Melissa Urban
Whole30 Co-Founder and CEO

ACKNOWLEDGMENTS

To be fair, this should more accurately be titled "A List of People I Am Forever Indebted to," because "Acknowledgments" just doesn't cut it. It's true: I owe a very serious debt of gratitude to so many people. There are those who not only gave me the opportunity to write this book but also helped me turn it into the very best version that it could possibly be. To borrow from the late, great Tupac Shakur, polishing the original form of this book was kind of like "trying to make a dollar out of 15 cents."

Melissa Urban, thank you for creating such an important program and continuing to foster its growth with unbridled enthusiasm. Not only have you produced remarkable resources and cultivated an incredible community for Whole30'ers, but you've also built a platform where people like me are able to share our passion and amplify our impact. Thank you for championing me, this book, and the message it carries with it. To the entire team at Whole30, who have believed in me from very early on, thank you as well.

To Lisa Grubka, my literary agent, thank you for emailing me that fateful day. You didn't know it, but your letter came at a pivotal time in my life. Thank you for your hard work and continued guidance over these past couple years. Thank you also to the team at Fletcher and Co. for making a very complex process seem easy.

To Justin Schwartz, my editor at Houghton Mifflin Harcourt, thank you for your belief in this book and your patience with its rookie author as it came together. Your impeccably sharp editorial skills and attention to detail are unmatched. I am extremely thankful to have learned a great deal from you, not least the art of properly writing a recipe. To the team at HMH and everyone who played a role in bringing this book to life, from editing and designing to marketing and PR, thank you for helping to make this dream a reality.

To Andrea Magyar and the team at Penguin Canada, thank you for bringing this book home to the North and for your work on its Canadian cover.

To my dream team—Donna Griffith, my incredibly talented photographer, and Laura Branson, my prop stylist extraordinaire—thank you for taking on this project. You brought these recipes to life and captured them in a beautiful way that no one else could. To Lisa Daly, thank you for working your magic behind the scenes and always lending a helping hand.

To Alex Snodgrass, Michelle Tam, Laura Vitale, Connor Carrick, Kirsten Buck, Teri Turner, and Diala Canelo, thank you for lending your words and support to this book. I am grateful for the friendships we've built.

To my wife, Catalina, you are my compass. When I feel lost, you always point me in the right direction. This book, and the blog that it is an extension of, would not be possible without your boundless encouragement and unconditional support. Thank you for believing in me and all my crazy ideas over the years. Whether I was pursuing a Ph.D. in medieval art and architectural history, a harebrained tech startup, or a food blog, you've had my back from day one. Thank you for tasting every single recipe with sheer scrutiny, for your brutal honesty when things didn't taste good, and for your help with washing Himalayan-size mountains of dishes. Most of all, I thank you for being the most incredible mother to Sofia.

To my daughter, Sofia, to whom this book is dedicated, you are my world. I want you to know that being your papa is my number-one priority and everything else comes second. No matter how busy life gets, I will always be there for you. You are so incredibly smart, resilient, strong, generous, forgiving, kind, loving, beautiful, and funny. You fill me with such an immense amount of joy, love, optimism, and inspiration that I feel as though I can accomplish anything. I only hope to be able to instill those same feelings in you as you grow into the strong and powerful woman your mother and I know you will become. I am counting the days until we can cook together and dream up all kinds of delicious recipes. I am forever grateful and proud to be your father.

To my parents, Dianna and Yakov, I didn't fully understand it as a kid, but I now realize all that you sacrificed so that we wouldn't have to. Thank you for being brave enough to move to Canada with no money, no ability to speak English, and no job prospects, all so that we could have a better life. Thank you for believing in me, even though you didn't always understand what it was I was doing. To my in-laws, Nicu and Codruta, thank you for accepting me into your family as though I was one of your own and for teaching me about your country, culture, and food. Your generosity, love, and support flow through the pages of this book.

Julian, you're the best big brother a guy could ask for. My love for food is, in very large part, thanks to you. You are probably the most adventurous eater I know and I thank you for always taking me along for the ride. To Marcela, thank you for introducing me to cassava, tapioca, and the best Paleo pancakes ever! Your endless support and enthusiasm for my blog and this book have not gone unnoticed. To Cosmin and Seira, thank you for your continued support over the years.

Most of all, thank you! Yes, YOU, the person reading this. It is because of your ceaseless support and encouragement over the years that this book exists. From the bottom of my heart and belly, I thank you. I hope that you use and abuse this book. That you love the recipes and never once feel as though you're restricted or are missing out on something. Most of all, I want you to know that it's never too late to make a lasting health change. If I can do it, so can you.

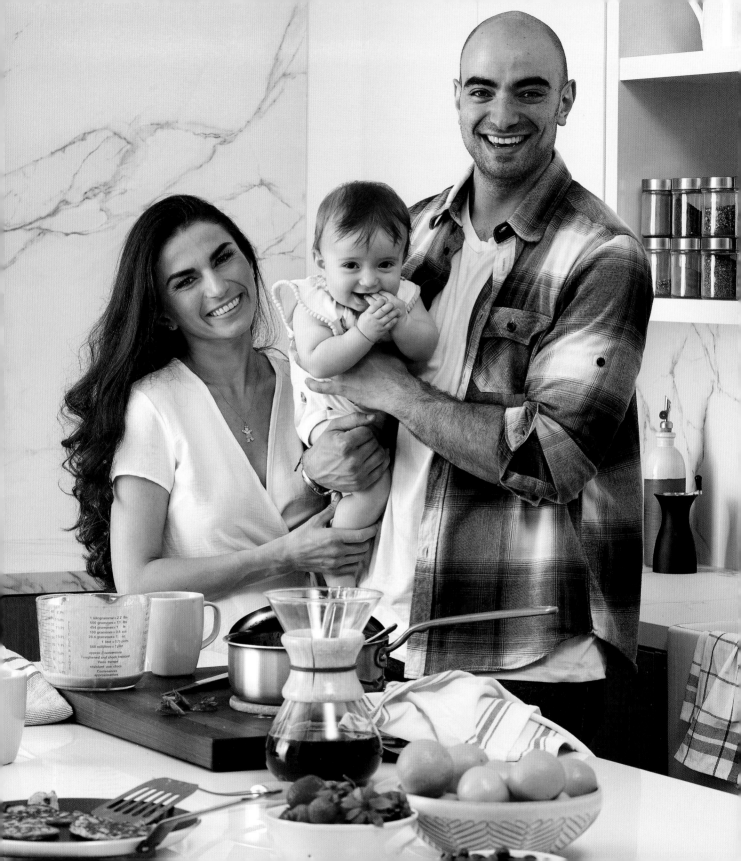

INTRODUCTION

DECEMBER 23, 2012. I hit my point of no return on the night of my twenty-seventh birthday, likely still drunk from the night out. After a lifetime of struggling with obesity, failed diets, and low self-esteem, I was fed up and decided to approach things differently. Instead of focusing on the numbers (pounds lost by days passed), which always brought me one step forward and two steps back, I wrote a list of ten qualitative resolutions that had nothing to do with weight:

1. Talk less, listen more
2. Think instead of reacting
3. Be honest
4. Don't wait until the new year to make more resolutions
5. Live a healthy life
6. Embrace all emotions
7. Practice moderation
8. Be environmentally conscious
9. Work harder at the things you love
10. Just breathe

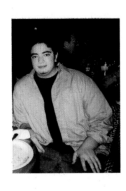

Most of the pictures I have from this time in my life are not ones I wanted taken. In fact, I hated having my picture taken. I was uncomfortable in my own skin. I would purposely wear several layers of clothing (even in the hottest months) and would try to slouch forward so that my clothes draped over me and concealed the shape of my body. I can't remember the exact date of this photo, but I remember it was taken at a Houston's restaurant in North Miami and that I ordered the full rack of ribs with a side of fries and coleslaw. I wouldn't be surprised if I ate the entire meal for a sense of comfort. I often thought the people around me were judging me, which led me to judge myself, continuing a downward spiral of self-loathing and more emotional eating.

I thought maybe, just maybe, if I approached health from a more holistic angle, rather than focusing on an arbitrary number on the scale or a date on the calendar, then perhaps I wouldn't get so hung up on failing at everything else, which only repeated a vicious, downward spiral. Heck, one of the resolutions was "Just breathe." So as long as I could stay alive, I'd be headed in the right direction.

I didn't want to wait until New Year's Day, only one week away, to get started. I was tired of waiting. I always let myself down and made excuses to delay things further. The very next morning, I began my health journey, determined to make a lasting change. I cleaned up my diet, ditched the booze, got a gym pass, started doing yoga, and began playing basketball with friends. By March, I was making strides with my fitness: I had managed to cut back on the junk food and booze, though not entirely, and even shed a couple pounds! Then, all of a sudden, I plateaued. No matter how hard I trained, meditated, or ran across the court, I wasn't making any more progress. I questioned where I went wrong and instinctively wanted to curl up with a cheeseburger and a six-pack of beer. I thought, *Well, Ronny, you had a good run while it lasted!* An all too familiar feeling of disappointment washed over me and I was ready to throw in the towel.

It was just around that time that one of my best friends invited my brother and me over for lunch. Roasted chicken thighs, sweet potatoes, and salad were on the menu. Admittedly, not the most exciting meal, but I found myself feeling full without the lethargy that always followed. My mind was blown. My friend said everything we ate was Paleo. *Paleo? What's Paleo?* I googled it. My phone was flooded with images of ripped guys and gals doing crazy stuff on pull-up bars and Olympic gymnastic rings. They were balancing barbells over their heads like strongmen in one picture and walking on their hands in another. I wanted to be one of those guys and gals! I wanted to do those things! I wanted to be Paleo! Most of the people preaching Paleo from the pulpits of the Internet weren't even calling it a "diet." They were calling it a "lifestyle." I wanted a "lifestyle"! From what I quickly gleaned, it promised to focus on real, simple, whole foods. The entire Paleo mentality meshed very well with my ten resolutions. It was a more holistic approach to eating and health than any "diet" I had ever encountered. With nothing to lose, I drank the Kool-Aid.

I was not prepared for what was about to happen. I already knew that junky processed foods were harmful, but Paleo also introduced me to the adverse health effects associated with foods I grew up believing were good for me: milk, cheese, oatmeal, white rice, whole wheat pasta, brown and multigrain bread! The more I read, the more I realized just how much damage I had done to myself over the years. All my childhood allergies, asthma, upset stomachs, headaches, back pain, lethargy, belly rolls, and cravings were explained. Everything became so clear. I felt like Neo standing in the hallway after seeing the Matrix!

Within a few months of following a Paleo lifestyle, the pounds had melted away. I grew stronger, faster, and more flexible. I inhaled deep, fulfilling, delicious breaths of air, something I had always struggled with from childhood asthma. I was finally starting to feel comfortable in my own skin. I regained confidence and couldn't believe my physical and psychological transformation. All the while, I cooked and ate delicious food. So delicious that I never once stopped to think that I was on a "diet."

It was within Paleo's fundamental principles (prioritizing vegetables, high-quality meats and seafood, nuts and seeds, and some fruit) that I saw new opportunities to be creative in the kitchen and nurture my passion for cooking and feeding people. In the summer of 2015, my wife and a group of close friends persuaded me to start a dedicated Instagram account to share photos of my meals with others. Every now and then, a friend would call me for a recipe. Sometimes I'd spend between 30 minutes and an hour walking them through their dinner as they cooked it on the other end of the line. It was fun, and I loved the idea that I was introducing someone else to Paleo. It was also a limiting and not very effective use of time. To make my life easier, another one

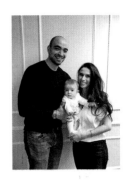

Though I'm far from perfect and continue to work on myself every day, much of the progress I've made in rehabilitating my body and relationship with food is thanks to my wife, Catalina. She has been with me through thick and thin, literally and figuratively. She is my biggest supporter, motivator, and moral compass. Without her continued encouragement, I don't think I would be where I am today. On December 23, 2018, the same day as my birthday, she gave birth to our daughter, Sofia. Just like her mom, Sofia inspires me to stay healthy, both physically and mentally, no matter how difficult it sometimes seems.

of my best friends suggested I start a blog. "What's a blog?" I asked. A couple days later, he built one for me (he's wicked smart) so that I could share full recipes, photos, and cooking tips and tricks.

Shortly after I began my blog, CookPrimalGourmet.com, I discovered Whole30 through Instagram. The program resonated with what I knew to be true of Paleo and I deeply related to the stories of its cofounder, Melissa Urban, and its millions of alumni. I often say that I completed my first round of Whole30 without even knowing it because I had been eating such a strict Paleo diet already. It wasn't until my first official round of Whole30, though, that I was able to really evaluate my relationship with food, thanks in large part to the Whole30 program literature, which helped me understand the true goals of the plan.

I learned a lot of lessons that month. First and foremost, that with a couple of years of clean eating under my belt, I was much better at identifying triggers and foods that don't sit well with me, but I was still far from perfect. I also realized that I still relied heavily on certain foods for comfort, to pass the time when I was bored, or just because I wanted to taste something. I live to eat, not eat to live. I am also an "at risk" eater, and likely always will be: at risk of falling off the wagon and back into old, unhealthy habits. When it comes to food, I have a very, very hard time having "just one" of anything worth having, be it a slice of pizza, a sushi roll, a cold beer, or a glass of scotch. What can I say? I love it all, and I'm very generous with my love! Sadly, the foods I loved growing up didn't love me back.

Over the past four or five years, CookPrimalGourmet.com has not only become a creative outlet for me and a way to share my recipes, but it has also grown into a platform that inspires others on their own health journeys. I don't ever take it for granted that people are willing to invest their time, energy, and money to make one of my recipes. I also take great pride in knowing that when people cook my recipes, they not only discover that healthy food can taste amazing, but they are also nourishing themselves, their families, and their friends without feelings of restriction, deprivation, or hunger.

The Primal Gourmet Cookbook is the first in what I hope will be a long line of cookbooks that prove *it's not a diet if it's delicious.*

Culinary Identity

In the process of writing this book, I thought very long and hard about culinary identity and whether I even have one. After all, I'm not a trained or professional chef. The extent of my culinary education is a half-day cooking class I took in Chiang Mai, Thailand, with a man named Basil.

For months on end, I spent every waking minute contemplating what kind of recipes would fill the pages of my very first cookbook. Should it be like a fine-tuned restaurant, where all the dishes fit tidily into a box labeled "French," "Italian," "Mexican," or "Greek"? Would my box have to be labeled "Russian"? Or, more accurately, "Canadian born to Lithuanian and Moldovan Jewish immigrants who just found it easier to say they were from Russia"? Does a cook's culinary identity have to align with their cultural, religious, or socioeconomic identity? The more I thought about it, the more I realized that my culinary identity is most largely informed by my family and the city I grew up in, Toronto. If I wasn't eating my mama's Matzo Ball Soup (page 77), my father's Pan-Fried Lamb Chops with Papa's Herby Ketchup (page 146), or my babushka Bronia's Borscht (page 105), I was out with my brother and friends scarfing down piping-hot bowls of Vietnamese pho, sweating over big plates of spicy Jamaican jerk chicken, stuffing my face with Lebanese shawarma and toum, enjoying Portuguese churrasco at least once a week, and loosening my belt after all-you-can-eat Indian feasts.

Toronto, with over 51 percent of its inhabitants born somewhere else and more than 250 nationalities represented in its population, is the world's most multicultural city. Such an incredible mosaic of cultures, religions, and ethnicities not only means there's an incredible variety of delicious foods available, but it also brings together people from all walks of life. I consider myself extremely fortunate to have been born and raised in Toronto. Its diversity and inclusivity are the primary reasons you'll find such a vast array of cultural influences in my recipes. I would like to make it clear, though, that my goal is never to pilfer, misrepresent, or subvert foods rooted in any person's or group's cultural heritage. On the contrary—I want to honor and engage with them in an effort to learn, experience, and savor cuisines and cultures other than my own. This is the exact same reason my wife and I travel as much as we do.

I understand that many of the dishes in this book are not my stories to tell and that I take certain liberties when it comes to how I prepare them. As a result, notions of authenticity and tradition often end up hanging in the balance. At the same time, I want to re-create and share delicious recipes in accessible and healthy ways so that they can be enjoyed by everyone, particularly those with food sensitivities or allergies. Sometimes that means replacing essential ingredients, as I do in my Fauxsole Verde con Pollo (page 66). Other times it means omitting things altogether, like the pita bread in my Sabich Platter (page 28). If my adaptations of these recipes offends you, then please accept my sincerest apologies in advance. It was not my intention. On the contrary, my goal has always been to use food as a way to bring people together, not separate them.

Paleo vs. Whole30

Unless specified otherwise, the recipes in this book are either Paleo-friendly or Whole30-compliant. This is a much easier way of saying they are gluten-free, dairy-free, grain-free, legume-free, refined sugar–free, and alcohol-free. They prioritize vegetables, high-quality meats and seafood, nuts and seeds, and some fruit. Some of the recipes are even keto-friendly, but I have to admit this is only by coincidence—I didn't set out to develop keto recipes. Only three recipes are not Paleo or Whole30: Creamy Hummus with Spiced Chickpeas (page 222), Moroccan Lamb Stew (page 134), and Matzo Ball Soup (page 77). The first two contain chickpeas, a legume. And the last one uses packaged matzo meal, made from ground, unleavened bread that is traditionally eaten during the Jewish holiday Passover (though in my mother's house, we ate it at every single holiday, Jewish or otherwise). I chose to include these recipes because they're delicious and easy to prepare. I love chickpeas and eat them on occasion, and as far as things to eat during life after Whole30, they're very good options.

While Paleo and Whole30 have a great deal in common, there are a few key differences I'd like to highlight.

The Whole30 program was designed and intended to be used as a thirty-day self-experiment. For thirty days, participants eliminate foods from their diet that are known to be generally harmful in an attempt to identify specific sensitivities and triggers. Paleo, on the other hand, is not restricted to a set time period and, ideally, can be the way you eat for the rest of your long, healthy life.

Whole30 is a set of black-and-white rules that are clearly structured and articulated. Paleo is a road map with shades of gray, and people interpret it in a variety of ways.

Paleo, for the most part, advises against the consumption of white potatoes; refined seed oils, such as sunflower oil; and certain vegetables, such as green beans. These are all permitted during a round of Whole30, with the exception that sunflower oil should only be consumed as a last resort, such as when you're dining out and the restaurant didn't bother to stock up on avocado oil to sauté your chicken.

Whole30 does not permit the consumption of "Paleofied" baked goods, junk foods, and treats. While things like Marcela's Paleo Pancakes (page 23) and Cassava Flour Tortillas (page 226) are Paleo and technically made with Whole30-friendly ingredients, they are not Whole30-compliant. The Whole30 term for these foods is SWYPO (Sex with Your Pants On). They're good, but nowhere near as good as the real thing. The purpose of excluding these foods during your round of Whole30 is to disconnect and rehabilitate the mental and emotional connection you may have to certain things, like a burger on a fluffy keto bun masquerading as the real deal. However, SWYPO foods might be something you want to try reintroducing in moderation once you've completed the program and moved into the Food Freedom stage, or life after Whole30.

In her book, *Food Freedom Forever*, Melissa Urban provides Whole30ers with the tools they'll need to live a healthy life after their thirty-day self-experiment. Because everyone is different, it's up to the individual to assess his or her personal relationship with food, be it physical or emotional, and determine what foods should be omitted entirely, what can be enjoyed in moderation, and what can be made part of a daily or weekly routine. Keep in mind, there is no one-size-fits-all solution to this, and basing your decisions on someone else's experience and routine is a recipe for disaster. I know from years of personal development that what works for others does not necessarily work for me. For example, it's very difficult for me to have just one serving of my Miracle Fish and Chips (page 178). I have to remind myself that even though it's a much healthier grain-free and gluten-free version of the greasy, deep-fat-fried fish and chips I grew up eating, it's still very calorie- and carbohydrate-dense and probably not healthy to eat in excess. It's also definitely not a step in the right direction when it comes to establishing a healthier relationship with food. Foods that have this kind of effect, ones that are very difficult to stop eating once you start, are referred to as "Food with No Brakes" by the folks at Whole30.

I also think it's important to note that working toward Food Freedom doesn't just have to apply to dealing with specific foods or drinks. It can also mean identifying the fact that eating a breakfast with whole, nutrient-dense foods is something that helps curb cravings and will likely set you up to make better food choices throughout the day.

For more information on SWYPO, Food Freedom, and all things Whole30, you can visit Whole30.com or pick up any of their printed resources. I have no doubt they'll do a better job of explaining it than me.

Grass-Fed, Organic, and Other Considerations

In a perfect world, where budget and availability are no concern, I would be exclusively eating grass-fed beef, lamb, and venison; organic, pasture-raised chickens and eggs; wild-caught seafood; heritage-breed, humanely raised pork; and organic fruits and vegetables. Alas, that is not the case.

I do, however, make a concerted effort to source the best possible ingredients my budget can afford. Sometimes that means making compromises. When it comes to produce, I do my best to purchase according to the Environmental Working Group's Clean 15 and Dirty Dozen lists. Every year the EWG comes out with a list of fruits and vegetables that regularly exhibit higher-than-normal pesticide levels, which they label the "Dirty Dozen." The EWG recommends purchasing organic versions of the Dirty Dozen. On the other hand, foods that show lower pesticide levels (and that you don't necessarily need to buy organic) are labeled the "Clean 15." I prefer to save money by purchasing conventional Clean 15 fruits and vegetables, and instead put the money toward buying high-quality meat that is humanely raised (whether that means grass-fed, organic, or wild-caught, when available). Not only do these proteins taste better, I know that I'm supporting businesses that are trying to change the food system for the better.

Getting Started

ESSENTIAL KITCHEN EQUIPMENT

I should make one thing very clear: Even though I refer to the following items as "essential," you don't *really need* any of them. My grandmother never used anything other than a paring knife and a beat-up old nonstick stockpot, and she could cook me under the table with her eyes closed.

Nevertheless, there is a certain level of joy that comes from cooking with tools, utensils, and gadgets that are thoughtfully and beautifully designed with quality and function in mind. Just try slicing through a tomato with a sharp Japanese blade, and you'll never want to go back to that janky hand-me-down knife your mom gave you before you left for college.

Since there's absolutely no way for me to know everyone's individual budget, I've listed the things I think should be in every home kitchen, regardless of skill level. It will be up to you to do some research when it comes to brands. Luckily, I have some articles on CookPrimalGourmet.com that can point you in the right direction.

Small Appliances

Food processor
Blender
Immersion blender
Slow cooker
Pressure cooker (electronic or stovetop)
Espresso maker (none of the recipes in this book actually requires an espresso maker, but I still think every home should have one)

Knives

7- or 8-inch chef's knife
3- or 4-inch paring knife
5-inch utility knife *or* 8-inch serrated (bread) knife

Cookware

8-inch nonstick pan *exclusively* for omelets

10-inch nonstick pan

12-inch nonstick pan

12-inch cast-iron or carbon-steel skillet

5-quart or 12-inch stainless-steel sauté pan

3-quart stainless-steel saucepan

5½-quart or larger Dutch oven

6-quart or larger stainless-steel stockpot with stainless-steel steamer insert

13 × 9-inch rimmed baking sheet

13 × 9-inch stainless-steel roasting pan or ceramic roasting dish (heavy-gauge stainless steel has the benefit of being stovetop-safe)

Utensils and Other Things

Large, edge-grain wooden cutting board

Large silicone cutting board (for raw meat and fish)

Medium wooden or silicone cutting board for smaller tasks

13 × 9-inch wire rack

Metal tongs

Balloon whisk

Rasp grater

Vegetable Y-peeler

Julienne peeler

Spiralizer

Liquid measuring cup

Set of dry measuring cups

Set of measuring spoons

Digital scale

Stainless-steel mixing bowls in a variety of sizes

Instant-read digital meat thermometer

Ladle

Wooden spoon

Silicone spatula

Pepper mill with adjustable grind setting

Box grater

Salad spinner

Japanese mandoline

Spider (strainer)

Colander

Fine-mesh sieve

Clear glass food storage bowls with lids in a variety of sizes

TABLE SALT

WINDSOR COARSE KOSHER SALT

SEL GRIS

HIMALAYAN PINK SALT

MALDON SEA SALT

FLEUR DE SEL

FINE SEA SALT

DIAMOND CRYSTAL KOSHER SALT

SPICES

Spice is the variety of life. Or is it "variety is the spice of life"? Either way, you're gonna need some spices!

One of the easiest and healthiest ways to add flavor to your food without extra calories is with dried herbs and spices. It should be every household's top priority to build a well-rounded spice pantry and to store them in airtight, widemouthed containers, so that you preserve freshness and can easily fit measuring spoons into them.

You don't necessarily have to buy spices in bulk. In fact, I don't recommend this, especially not from stores that sell their dried herbs and spices in bulk from giant vats that are exposed to oxygen—and thousands of people's hands! Dried herbs and spices don't generally expire, but they will go stale and lose their flavor over time, so you might be better off sourcing them in smaller, prepackaged quantities and using them up as quickly as possible. To save money, look for dried herbs and spices sold in recyclable packages instead of in those small glass jars. You pay a premium for the container; instead, use the money you save to buy small, widemouthed jars that you can easily refill and that are better suited to your pantry or spice drawer.

TYPES OF SALT AND WHEN TO USE THEM

Kosher salt is my salt of choice because of the size of its crystals, and it's less salty by volume than fine sea salt. I store my salt in a crock or in a small, widemouthed container with a lid, and unless I'm measuring things for a recipe, I just grab some salt with my fingers and season by eye and touch. Kosher salt is great because the relatively large crystals stay between my fingers, as opposed to fine sea salt, which tends to fall through the cracks like grains of sand.

Unless otherwise specified, all the recipes in this book were cooked with and repeatedly tested using Diamond Crystal kosher salt. This is not a paid endorsement, though I kind of wish it were. I like Diamond Crystal brand because it's not expensive, it's an ideal coarseness, and its rounder crystals tend to stick to things like protein and vegetables a bit better than other brands. Please note that if you're using a different brand of kosher salt, your recipes may either be saltier or not salty enough, depending on the coarseness of the salt. You might be able to find comparisons and substitution guides online if you can't find any Diamond Crystal kosher salt.

As always, there's a time and place for everything, and sometimes I use other types of salt. For example, I season my 30-Mississippi Mayonnaise (page 230) with fine sea salt because the finer crystals dissolve more easily into the sauce. I sometimes garnish finished dishes like roasted vegetables with a touch of flaky sea salt, such as Maldon, for a pop of salt and crunch.

There are myriad salts to choose from, and each has pros and cons. The good news is almost all salt, except maybe iodized table salt, does not go stale or bland. Especially if you store it in airtight containers. So feel free to stock up on all the varieties and play around with different tastes, textures, sizes, and colors!

Kosher Salt

Ideal for everyday cooking. Use it to season proteins, vegetables, sauces, and everything in between. It is the backbone for building flavor.

Fine Sea Salt

Because of its finer crystals, fine sea salt is very salty by volume. If a recipe calls for 1 teaspoon kosher salt, you may only need about half that amount of fine sea salt. You can cook with it and use it to season proteins, vegetables, and sauces, but keep the overall volume in mind.

Coarse Sea Salt

Slightly coarser than kosher salt, depending on the brand, and only slightly less suited to everyday cooking. The crystals won't stick to things as easily as kosher salt, which may result in unevenly seasoned food and some wasted salt.

Flaky Sea Salt

There's only one thing I love more than my kosher salt, and that's flaky sea salt! Brands like Maldon, Jacobsen Salt Co., and smaller boutique companies are producing fantastic salts. Some of the crystals look like tiny pyramids or precious gems! Because they tend to be more expensive, I recommend saving them for special occasions and using them as finishing salts. They're great when you want a touch more saltiness in addition to some texture.

Himalayan Pink Salt

Often touted as the world's purest form of salt, Himalayan pink salt is mined near the foothills of the Himalaya Mountains in the Punjab region of Pakistan. It usually comes in large crystals like rock salt and needs to be freshly ground. It can be used in everyday cooking, but like fine sea salt, it is saltier by volume than kosher salt.

Sel Gris

Recognizable by its relatively coarse crystals and light-gray hue, *sel gris*, French for "gray salt," has long been harvested off the coast of France. The gray color is imparted by the clay salt pans that come into contact with the salt before it is harvested. Celtic Sea Salt is one brand of *sel gris* that, despite the name, is similarly harvested off the coast of France, as well as other locations, like Guatemala. *Sel gris is* usually sold in coarse crystals and is saltier by volume than kosher salt. If you're going to use it, do so sparingly and as a finishing salt over cooked proteins and vegetables.

Fleur de Sel

Whereas Celtic Sea Salt (and other types of *sel gris*) is harvested from clay salt pans after seawater has evaporated, fleur de sel ("flower of salt" in French) forms in paper-thin crystals on the surface of salt ponds and is harvested by hand using wooden rakes. It is used almost exclusively as a garnish, similar to flaky sea salt, and adds a nice pop of flavor and texture to cooked proteins and vegetables.

Rock Salt

Perhaps the only times you'll cook with rock salt are if you decide to grill *picanha* (rump steak) the traditional Brazilian way, bake a whole fish in a salt crust, or need to serve oysters on the half shell on a bed of salt.

Table Salt

Table salt is mined from underground salt deposits and is highly processed to remove minerals that add flavor and color to the salt. It is usually sold in very fine crystals and fortified with iodine, which was added around the 1920s to help prevent iodine deficiencies. This may be a good or a bad thing. I'm not a registered dietician, nutritionist, or doctor (at least not a medical one), so I leave it up to you to do some more research. As far as cooking goes, it's very salty by volume, so keep that in mind if using it in recipes.

WHOLE30-COMPLIANT AND PALEO-FRIENDLY OILS AND WHEN TO USE THEM

Extra-Virgin Olive Oil

Buying extra-virgin olive oil is very much like choosing a great bottle of wine. Most people just look at the label or the price before making a decision. The fact is, not all olive oils are created equal, and quality makes a big difference in flavor, nutrition, and cost.

First and foremost, look for an oil that is labeled "extra-virgin." This is the highest designation of quality for olive oils. "Cold-pressed" is another sign of high quality, and it means that the olives were kept below 80°F (27°C) during the extraction process, thereby preserving antioxidants like tocopherols and polyphenols in the oil. Likewise, the designation "first-pressed" means the oil was extracted from olives that were crushed and pressed only once (repeated

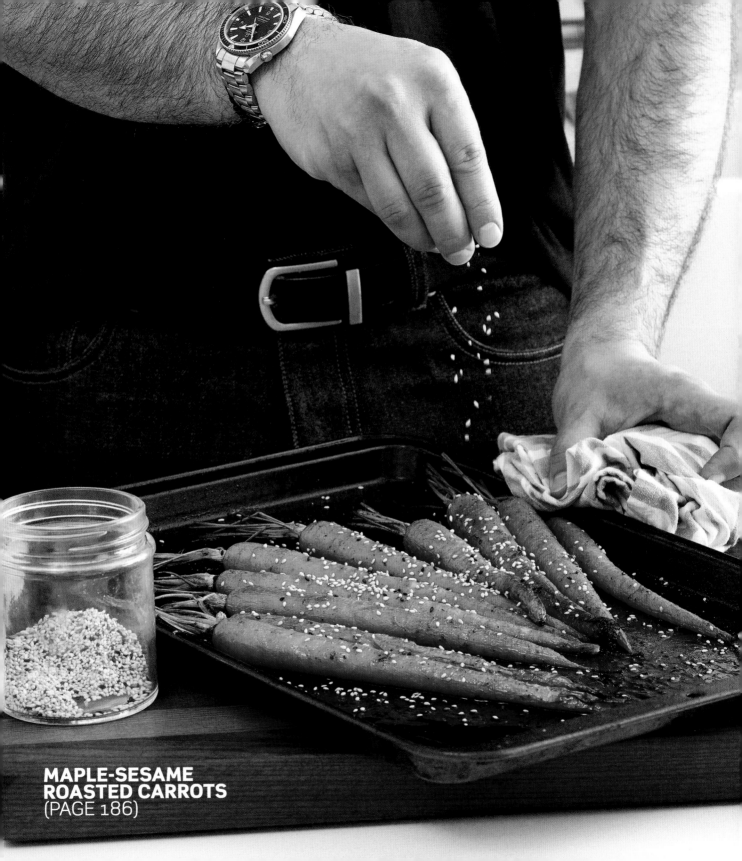

**MAPLE-SESAME
ROASTED CARROTS**
(PAGE 186)

pressings result in a lower-quality oil). It's important to know that the International Olive Council requires true extra-virgin olive oils to be first cold-pressed. So if you see one of these terms without the other, be wary. Likewise, if you don't see the words *extra-virgin*, such as when you buy "extra-light" or "light-tasting" olive oil, the oil has likely been stripped of valuable nutrients and flavor, and at that point, you might as well buy sunflower oil.

Once you've identified a cold-pressed extra-virgin olive oil, you'll want to make sure it comes in a dark glass or steel bottle. The container should be opaque, because light will cause the oil to denature over time. If you can find a bottle with a harvest, a bottled-on date, and/or an expiration date, those are also good signs that the manufacturer is disclosing freshness.

Country of origin and location of bottling are also important considerations. Look for oils that are made from single-origin olives and bottled in the region where those olives were grown, such as Greece, California, Tunisia, or Italy. After all, olives grown in Greece but bottled in New Jersey will undoubtedly lose some freshness along the way and the oil's flavor profile will reflect that.

Despite what you may have heard, "light" or "extra-light" olive oil is not a good source of fat. As mentioned, it has been stripped of its nutrients through processing and heat. In the Paleo and Whole30 communities, "light" olive oil is commonly used to make homemade mayonnaise, aioli, dipping sauces, and salad dressings because of its neutral flavor and low cost. Personally, I prefer to use a refined avocado oil when I want something neutral in flavor. Not only is it a healthier choice, but it can also be used for cooking.

Having said all of the above, I understand that cost is always a consideration, so just be sure to purchase the best quality product your budget can afford. The good news is, places like Costco and Trader Joe's sell organic extra-virgin olive oil for a great price. So get out there and start hunting!

I use extra-virgin olive oil in my day-to-day cooking. It goes into my salad dressings and vinaigrettes, sauces like Classic Salsa Verde (page 237), and sometimes my roasts. I also use it when sautéing at lower temperatures when I want to impart some flavor and color into the dish. I've read some conflicting studies about extra-virgin olive oil's smoking point (the temperature at which an oil begins to smoke and burn), and maybe you have, too. Some studies indicate olive oil becomes chemically unstable and deteriorates even at low heat; others report that it is perfectly suited for moderately high temperature cooking of around 350°F, insofar as it is truly extra-virgin and rich in antioxidants. Clearly, I'll have to do some more research before siding with one conclusion over the other, and I encourage you to do the same.

Refined Avocado Oil

Next to extra-virgin olive oil, avocado oil is my main cooking fat. It's incredibly versatile, neutral in flavor and light in color, and it has a high smoking point, making it suitable for cooking at high temperatures. It can be used for everything from stir-fries to roasts to 30-Mississippi Mayonnaise (page 230) to Uncle Ronny's Salsa Verde (page 244) and everything in between. It's particularly good if you need an oil that won't impart any additional flavor, as extra-virgin olive oil would.

Coconut Oil

Coconut oil has a slightly sweet, aromatic, and coconutty flavor. It has a high smoking point, making it suitable for cooking at high temperatures, but the trade-off is that it imparts some flavor. Try using it in recipes that have complementary flavors, such as Thai curries, Asian stir-fries, Twice-Fried Plantains (page 218), Sweet Plantains (Maduros) (page 210), or anywhere else you want to add coconut flavor. I'm told it's also a great conditioner for your hair. I wouldn't know, because I'm bald.

Ghee

Like regular clarified butter, ghee is made by slowly heating butter in a pot until the milk solids can be removed. Whereas clarified butter usually involves skimming milk solids as they foam and rise to the surface, ghee is cooked for a longer period of time to allow for the milk solids to sink and brown before being taken out. The result is a slightly nuttier, richer-tasting, and more flavorful finished product that can be used as a Paleo-friendly and Whole30-compliant butter replacement. Use it to make everything from fried eggs to roasted potatoes to compound "butter," and to baste chicken, seafood, and steaks. Since the dairy solids have been removed from the butterfat, it also has a high smoking point and is suitable for cooking at high temperatures. For those with dairy allergies, it's important to note that although ghee is free of lactose, it still contains traces of dairy.

Grass-Fed Butter

Grass-fed butter is a delicious source of fat. Some people consider it Paleo-friendly and others don't, and it's not Whole30-compliant (though you can choose to include it after the program). I tend to use it sparingly, which makes it all the more special for me. Every so often, I'll sneak it into my Smoked Salmon Scramble (page 26) or some scrambled eggs. It's especially delicious blended into my morning coffee, along with collagen peptides and MCT oil. (There's a trademarked name for this beverage that I won't use for fear of infringement, but it's incredibly delicious and something I look forward to most mornings.)

BRAISING IN SLOW COOKERS AND PRESSURE COOKERS

Braising is a cooking technique that uses both dry and wet heats. It is ideal for tougher cuts of meat: the long cooking times break down the meat's connective tissue, and the addition of a liquid keeps the meat moist as it cooks. A protein (or vegetable) is seared or browned in a hot pan, then liquid is added, the heat lowered, and the dish is cooked until tender, either on the stovetop or in the oven. It is, by far, my favorite technique, and one I think every home cook should learn, not least because it allows you to transform less-coveted cuts of meat, which are usually more affordable than select cuts, into the most delicious, mouth-watering, fall-off-the-bone-tender finished products. Braises also usually taste even better the next day, so they're great for meal-prepping large batches.

A few recipes in this book call for braising, such as my Short Rib Ragù (page 103), Ancho-Braised Lamb Shanks (page 137), Slow Cooker Mojo Pork (page 150), Curry Lamb and Potatoes (page 139), Zharkoe (page 113), and Pomegranate Braised Lamb Shanks (page 152). Each of these can be cooked in a slow cooker, pressure cooker, or in a pot on the stovetop or in the oven; the technique is virtually identical. Regardless of which method you use, I recommend beginning each braise by browning the protein (or vegetable) in a pot on the stovetop. This small step helps develop a significant amount of flavor on the protein and in the subsequent sauce, which should be started in the same pan by deglazing with a liquid.

In other words, if you want to make my Short Rib Ragù in your pressure cooker, don't just dump all the ingredients in, seal the lid, and hope for the best. Instead, take the time to brown the meat, sauté the vegetables, and deglaze the pan with the tomato sauce. Then, and only then, should you cook under high pressure. The same goes if you are using a slow cooker.

Using a pressure cooker for braising does, however, have some caveats. While you can cut down on cooking time by as much as three-quarters by using a pressure cooker, the flavor of the dish will likely not be as pronounced as something that has been braised on the stovetop or in the oven, and the sauce will not be concentrated. Why? Pressure cookers trap steam, which increases the pressure and heat in the pot. But because of that steam, pressure cookers don't allow any significant reduction or concentration of liquid in the pot. If anything, you'll usually notice more liquid in the pot after you cook something because juices will have rendered from the meat or vegetables. In contrast, cooking on the stovetop or in the oven allows excess moisture to evaporate, giving sauces the chance to reduce and their flavors to concentrate.

The good news is, there's a workaround! After pressure-cooking a protein such as my Ancho-Braised Lamb Shanks, transfer the cooked lamb to a bowl and cook the liquid in the pressure cooker using the SAUTÉ function until it has thickened into a sauce.

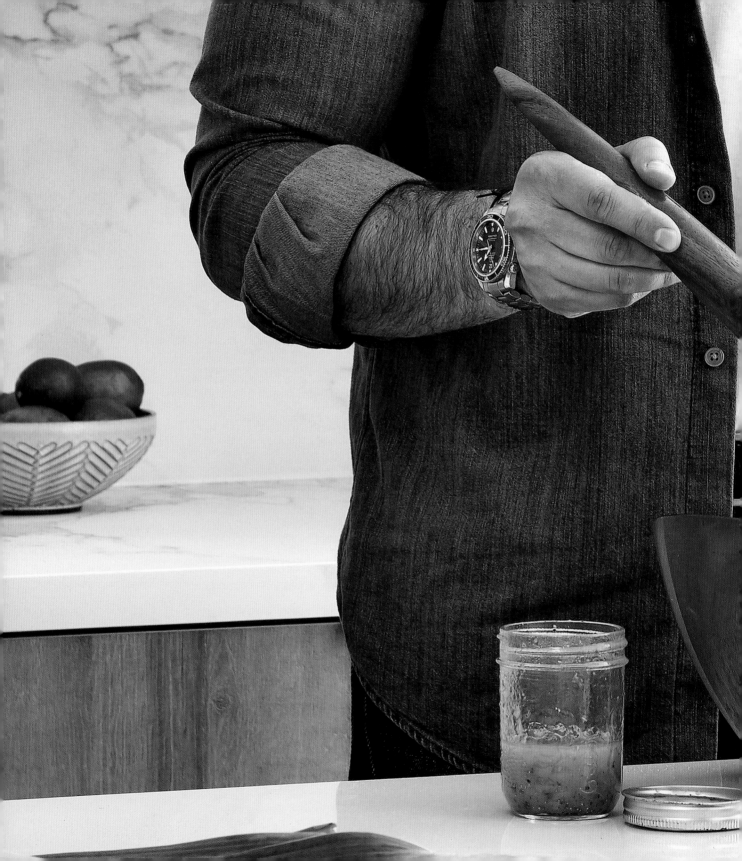

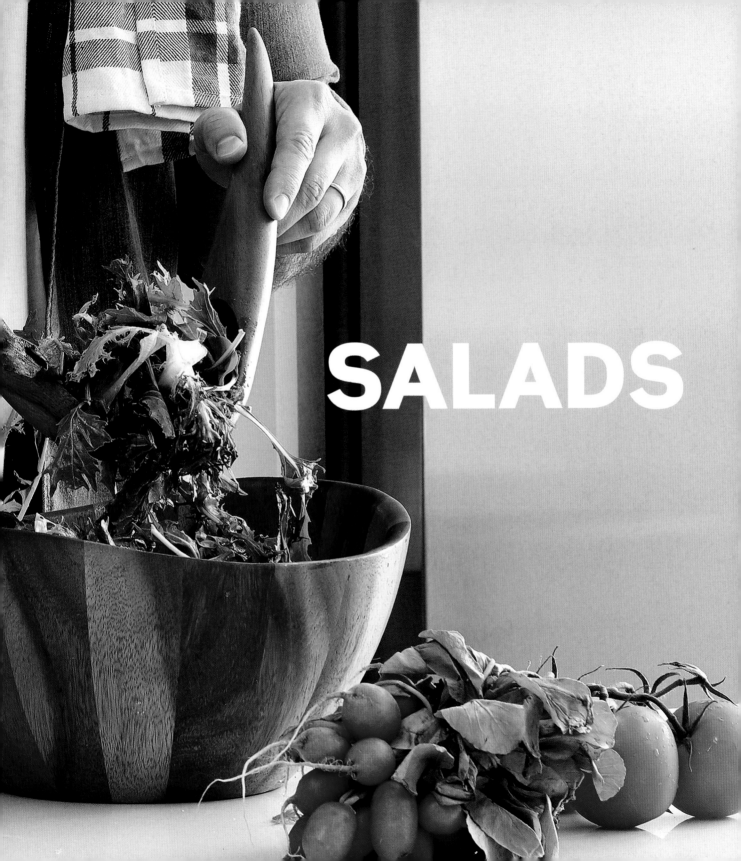

SALADS

CARAWAY CABBAGE COLESLAW

Gluten-Free

Dairy-Free

Whole30

Paleo

Grain-Free

Sugar-Free

Time: 50 minutes

½ cup 30-Mississippi Mayonnaise (page 230)

2 tablespoons apple cider vinegar

¾ teaspoon kosher salt

¼ teaspoon freshly ground black pepper

1 small head green cabbage (about 2 pounds), cored and thinly sliced using a food processor or mandoline

2 large carrots, shredded

1 red onion, thinly sliced

¼ cup fresh parsley leaves, finely chopped

1 tablespoon caraway seeds

Bring this coleslaw to your next cookout, and your friends and family won't be disappointed. The secret ingredient is caraway seeds, which add a subtle and unexpected flavor. Try serving it with my Jerk Chicken (page 55) or Jerk Ribs (page 142) for a Jamaican-inspired lunch or dinner.

In a small bowl, whisk together the mayonnaise, vinegar, ¼ teaspoon of the salt, and the pepper until smooth. Refrigerate until ready to use.

Put the cabbage in a large bowl and cover with cold water. Agitate the cabbage a bit with your hands, rinse well, and drain in a colander. Season the cabbage with the remaining ½ teaspoon salt and massage the salt into the cabbage with your hands. Let the cabbage drain for at least 15 minutes or up to 1 hour.

Squeeze as much moisture out of the cabbage as possible and transfer the cabbage back to the large bowl. Add the carrots, onion, parsley, caraway seeds, and the mayonnaise mixture. Toss everything to coat, cover with plastic wrap, and refrigerate for at least 30 minutes and up to 24 hours before serving to let the flavors come together.

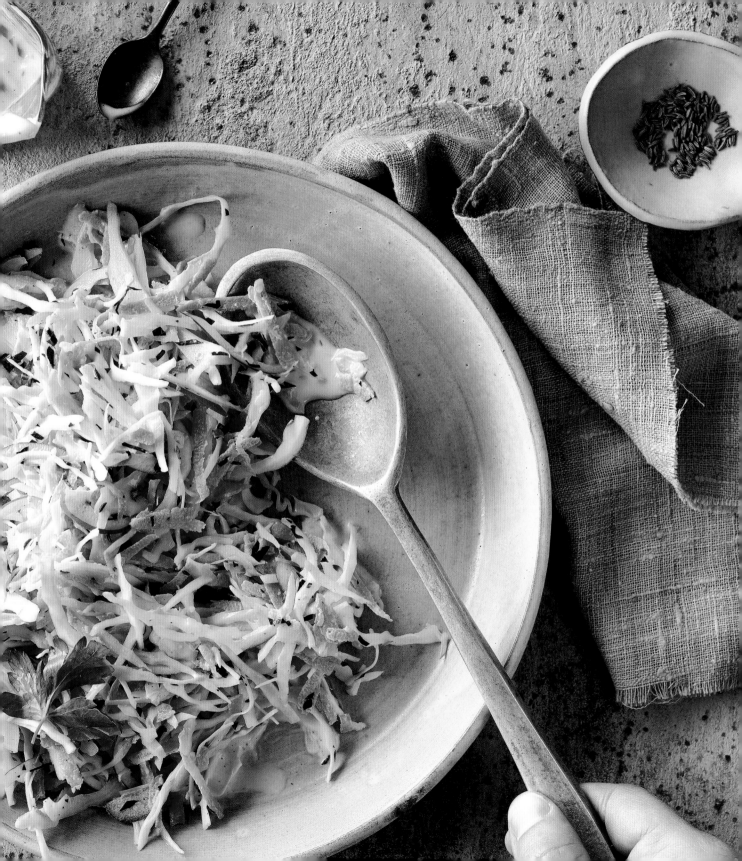

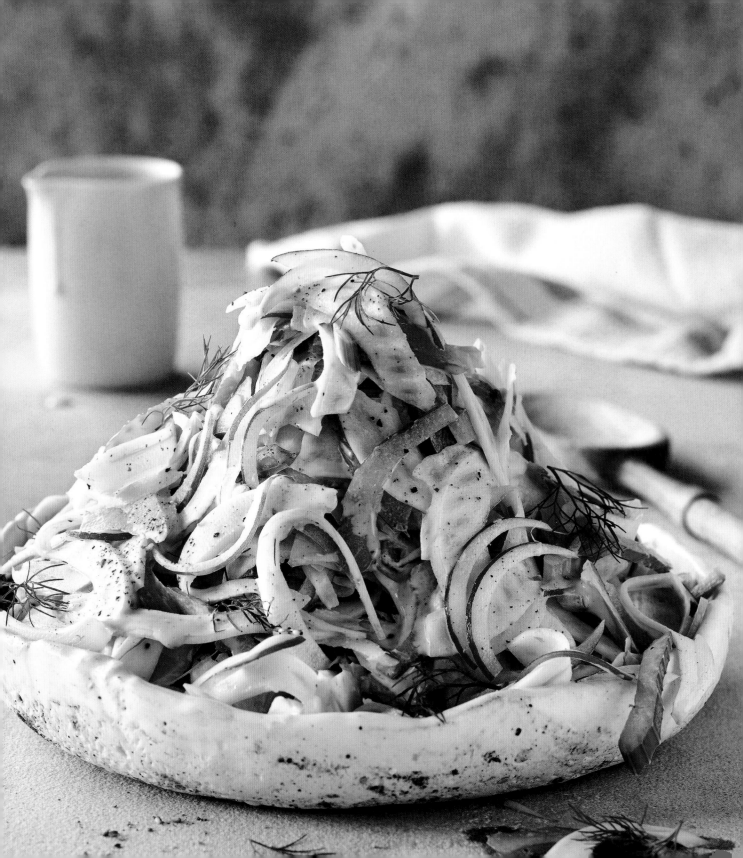

CREAMY FENNEL AND CELERY SLAW

Fennel and celery are two supremely underrated vegetables. They're extremely versatile in that they can be roasted, sautéed, or enjoyed raw. Here I bring together the two in a crisp and fresh coleslaw. Try serving it with my Chicken Schnitzel (page 40) for a next-level flavor combination. You can omit the honey if you're doing a round of Whole30. The slaw will have a bit more tang to it, but that's not necessarily a bad thing here.

In a large bowl, whisk together the mayonnaise, honey, vinegar, mustard, salt, and pepper until smooth. Add the fennel, celery, and onion. Toss to coat and let sit for 5 to 10 minutes before serving.

¼ cup 30-Mississippi Mayonnaise (page 230)

1 tablespoon honey (omit for Whole30)

1 tablespoon sherry vinegar

1 tablespoon Dijon mustard

¼ teaspoon kosher salt

⅛ teaspoon freshly ground black pepper

2 fennel bulbs, thinly shaved (a mandoline works great for this)

2 celery stalks, thinly sliced on an angle

1 small red onion, thinly sliced

Gluten-Free
Dairy-Free
Whole30, if modified
Keto-Friendly
Paleo
Grain-Free

Time: 15 minutes

CHOPPED SALAD

Gluten-Free

Dairy-Free

Whole30

Paleo

Grain-Free

Sugar-Free

Keto-Friendly

Time: 5 minutes

4 Persian cucumbers, diced

2 Roma (plum) tomatoes, diced

½ red onion, diced

¼ cup loosely packed fresh parsley leaves, finely chopped

2 tablespoons extra-virgin olive oil

1 tablespoon fresh lemon juice

2 teaspoons ground sumac

Kosher salt and freshly ground black pepper

You'll find versions of this chopped salad all throughout the Middle East and the Mediterranean, where each country tends to put its own spin on things. In Iran, dried or fresh mint is added, and it's called salad Shirazi. In Turkey, cooks often include bell peppers and scallions and chop the veggies a bit less finely, and call it *çoban salatasi*, meaning "shepherd's salad." You might also see similar versions referred to as Arabic salad, Palestinian salad, or Israeli salad, depending on where you're ordering it.

It is incredibly easy to prepare, uses only a few ingredients, and is very delicious. It's a fantastic side dish for just about any roasted or grilled protein you can imagine, and it's also very good alongside some hard-boiled eggs for breakfast. In fact, this chopped salad plays a key role in my Sabich Platter (page 28). Personally, I like to include a dash or two of ground sumac, which not only adds a hint of tartness, but also some color.

In a large bowl, combine the cucumbers, tomatoes, onion, parsley, olive oil, lemon juice, and sumac. Taste and season with salt and pepper as desired. Serve, or cover and refrigerate for 2 to 3 days.

KALE, ARUGULA, AND PEAR SALAD
WITH WALNUTS AND PROSCIUTTO

Everyone should have a good kale salad in their arsenal. It's healthy, easy to prepare, and a crowd-pleaser, and it always looks fancier than it actually is. This version is studded with arugula for some peppery bite, sliced pear for sweetness and texture, and walnuts for a nutty crunch. The salad is dressed with some May All Your Pain Be Champagne Vinaigrette before being draped with delicate slices of prosciutto di Parma. I love the dramatic effect of serving the salad to guests and having them peel back the slices of cured ham to reveal the ingredients beneath.

There are two secrets to making a great kale salad. First: Chop the leaves as finely as possible. Second: Massage the leaves with a tiny bit of extra-virgin olive oil and salt. This will help the kale's tough texture by significantly softening the leaves. It makes a huge difference in the finished product, so try not to skip this step.

In a large nonstick or stainless-steel skillet, toast the walnuts over medium heat, stirring occasionally, until golden brown and fragrant, 3 to 4 minutes. Transfer the nuts to a bowl or plate and set aside.

Use your hands to strip the kale leaves from their stems. Reserve the stems for Kale Stem Frittata (page 37). Transfer the leaves to a large bowl, drizzle them with the olive oil, and season with the salt. Use your hands to gently massage the oil and salt into the kale until the kale has softened slightly and is dark green in color and glistening from the oil, about 3 minutes.

Add the arugula and drizzle with the vinaigrette. Toss everything to coat and transfer to a serving platter.

Garnish with the pear and toasted walnuts and drape the prosciutto slices over the top. Serve immediately.

¼ cup coarsely chopped raw unsalted walnuts

1 pound curly kale (about 1 bunch)

1 teaspoon extra-virgin olive oil

¼ teaspoon kosher salt

1 cup arugula

¼ cup May All Your Pain Be Champagne Vinaigrette (page 252)

1 Bosc pear, cored and cut into ⅛-inch-thick slices

4 slices prosciutto di Parma

Gluten-Free

Dairy-Free

Whole30

Paleo

Grain-Free

Time: 15 minutes

FAUXTTOUSH

Gluten-Free
Dairy-Free
Whole30
Keto-Friendly
Paleo
Grain-Free
Sugar-Free

Time: 30 minutes

For the Vinaigrette:

¼ cup extra-virgin olive oil

Juice of ½ lemon

1 tablespoon red wine vinegar

1 garlic clove, finely chopped

1 teaspoon ground sumac

1 teaspoon dried parsley

¼ teaspoon kosher salt, plus more as needed

⅛ teaspoon freshly ground black pepper, plus more as needed

For the Salad:

2 heads romaine lettuce, coarsely chopped into 2-inch pieces

6 radishes, thinly sliced into rounds

3 Persian cucumbers, sliced into thin half-moons

2 vine-ripened tomatoes, cut into 1-inch pieces

½ red onion, thinly sliced

12 fresh mint leaves, thinly sliced

¼ cup loosely packed fresh parsley leaves, coarsely chopped

Fattoush is a Middle Eastern salad commonly made with mixed greens, cucumbers, tomatoes, onions, mint, parsley, and the secret ingredient: fried flatbread or pita. The salad is tossed in a tangy vinaigrette laced with ground sumac. Here I include everything except for the fried bread (hence "faux" in the title), which keeps things Paleo and Whole30-compliant. It's still incredibly delicious and makes for an excellent garden salad to accompany roasted or grilled meats or seafood.

MAKE THE VINAIGRETTE: In a mason jar, combine the olive oil, lemon juice, vinegar, garlic, sumac, parsley, salt, and pepper. Cover tightly with a lid and shake until combined. Taste and adjust the salt and pepper as desired.

MAKE THE SALAD: In a large bowl, combine the lettuce, radishes, cucumbers, tomatoes, onion, mint, and parsley. Drizzle the vinaigrette over the top and toss to coat. Let sit for 10 to 15 minutes before serving.

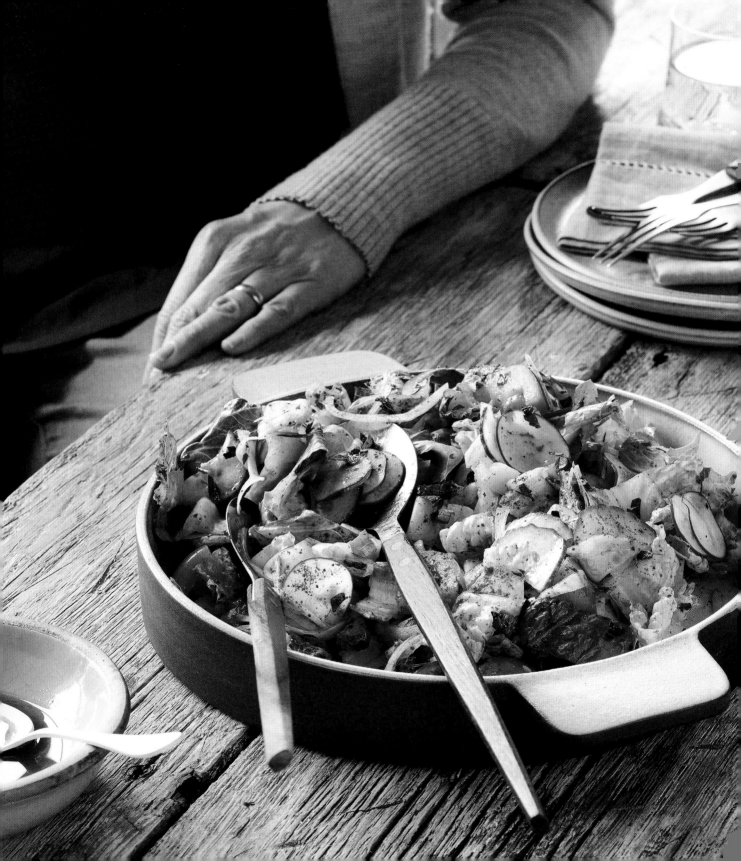

EVERYTHING-BUT-THE-BAGEL SALAD

Gluten-Free
Dairy-Free
Whole30
Keto-Friendly
Paleo
Grain-Free
Sugar-Free

Time: 25 minutes

2 large eggs

½ head iceberg lettuce, finely shredded, or 2 cups mixed greens

2 vine-ripened tomatoes, cut into 8 wedges

½ English cucumber, thinly sliced

1 avocado, cut into wedges

4 radishes, thinly sliced

½ small red onion, thinly sliced

4 ounces no-sugar-added smoked salmon

1 tablespoon capers packed in brine, drained

2 tablespoons extra-virgin olive oil

1 tablespoon fresh lemon juice

1 tablespoon Bagel Be Gone Seasoning (page 256)

Inspired by a famous spice mixture (for which I've shared a recipe on page 256), this salad has everything you could ever want on your Sunday afternoon bagel, minus the bagel. I like to serve it family-style with all the ingredients separated so people can pick and choose what they like in their salad. There's always that one person who just isn't crazy about capers!

This recipe serves two, but it can be easily adjusted to serve more people—just double (or triple) the ingredient quantities as needed.

Fill a large bowl with ice and water and set it nearby.

Bring a small pot of water to a boil over high heat. Using a slotted spoon, slowly lower the eggs into the water, being careful not to crack them on the bottom of the pot. Cook the eggs for exactly 12 minutes for hard yolks and whites. Transfer the eggs to the ice bath and let cool for at least 5 minutes.

Peel the eggs and slice them into quarters.

Arrange the eggs, lettuce, tomatoes, cucumber, avocado, radishes, onion, salmon, and capers side by side on a large serving platter. Drizzle the salad with the olive oil and lemon juice and sprinkle with the Bagel Be Gone Seasoning. Serve immediately.

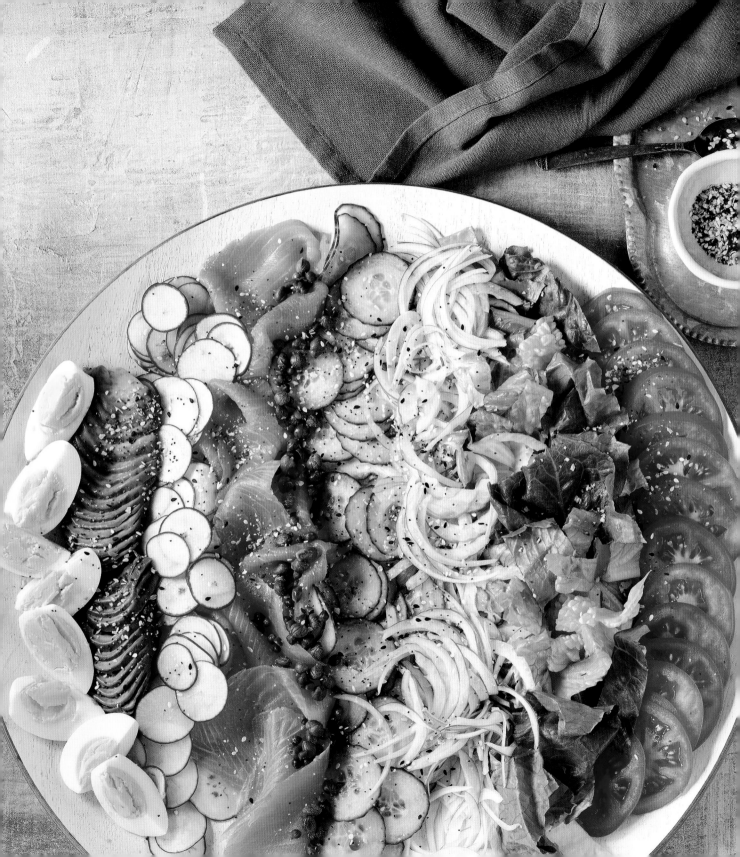

GRILLED SHRIMP COBB

Gluten-Free

Dairy-Free

Paleo

Grain-Free

Time: 30 minutes

4 large eggs

4 slices bacon

¾ pound raw jumbo shrimp (21/25 count), peeled and deveined

1 tablespoon Adobo Seasoning (page 254)

6 cups mixed greens

3 or 4 vine-ripened tomatoes, cut into 8 wedges each

1 large avocado, cut into wedges

½ small red onion, thinly sliced

¼ cup California Classic (Balsamic Vinaigrette) (page 248)

¼ cup coarsely chopped fresh dill

It's hard to beat an epic Cobb salad, and this one is no exception. It's loaded with seasoned grilled shrimp, crispy bacon, juicy tomatoes, creamy avocado, and hard-boiled eggs. Try drizzling it with my California Classic vinaigrette for the greatest salad of all time. OK, maybe that's an overstatement, but if you know me, you know I get excited about good salads.

Fill a large bowl with ice and water and set it nearby.

Bring a small pot of water to a boil over high heat. Using a slotted spoon, slowly lower the eggs into the water, being careful not to crack them on the bottom of the pot. Cook the eggs for exactly 6 minutes for soft-boiled runny yolks and cooked whites, or 12 minutes for firm yolks and whites. Transfer the eggs to the ice bath and let cool for at least 5 minutes.

Peel the eggs and slice them in half.

Place the bacon in a large nonstick skillet and set it over medium-high heat. Cook until the bacon is browned, about 5 minutes, then flip and cook until crispy, about 3 minutes more. Transfer the cooked bacon to a plate lined with paper towels to absorb excess grease. Pour off all but 2 tablespoons of the rendered fat from the skillet.

Once the bacon slices are cool enough to handle, chop them in half and set aside.

Return the skillet with the reserved bacon fat to medium-high heat. Add the shrimp, season with the Adobo Seasoning, and cook until they are pink and firm, 2 to 3 minutes per side.

Arrange the greens, shrimp, tomatoes, eggs, avocado, onion, and bacon on a large serving platter. Dress with the vinaigrette, garnish with the dill, and serve.

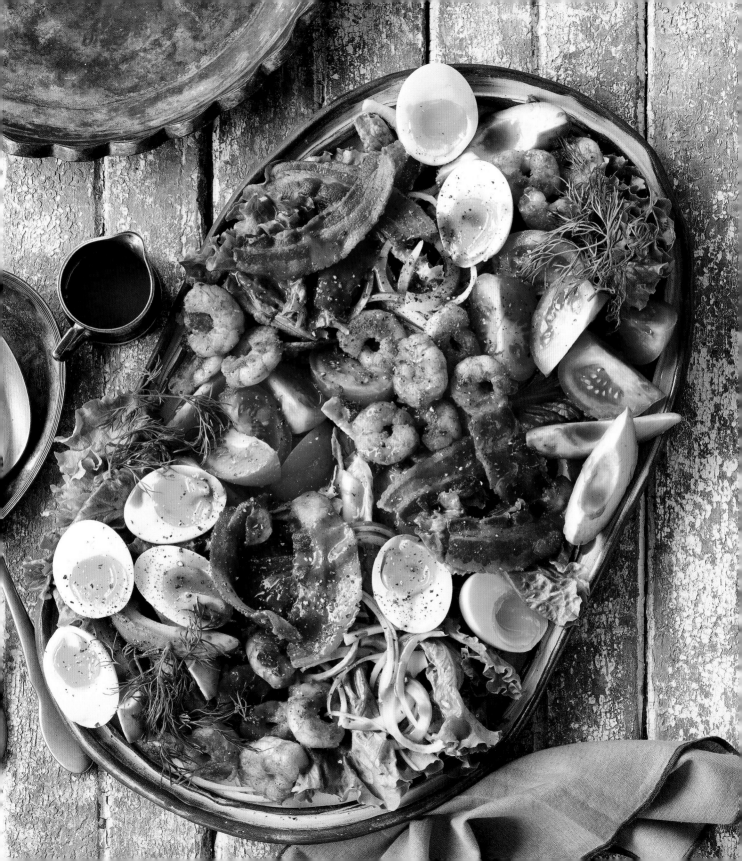

MEDITERRANEAN TUNA SALAD

Gluten-Free

Dairy-Free

Whole30

Keto-Friendly

Paleo

Grain-Free

Sugar-Free

Time: 10 minutes

1 (3-ounce) can chunk light tuna packed in water, drained

3 tablespoons extra-virgin olive oil

2 tablespoons fresh lemon juice

1 tablespoon finely chopped fresh parsley leaves

1 teaspoon capers packed in brine, drained

½ teaspoon red pepper flakes

¼ teaspoon dried oregano

¼ teaspoon freshly ground black pepper

3 cups mixed greens

¼ cup canned artichoke hearts packed in water, drained

1 vine-ripened tomato, cut into 8 wedges

1 Persian cucumber, thinly sliced

1 tablespoon finely chopped sun-dried tomatoes packed in olive oil, drained

At least twice a week, I find myself staring into the refrigerator and muttering, "We have nothing to eat." As a matter of fact, it happened this morning! The good news is, this Mediterranean tuna salad is a great contingency plan. It relies on pantry and refrigerator staples and comes together in less than 10 minutes. I usually allot one can of tuna per person, so feel free to double, triple, or quadruple the recipe according to how many servings you need.

In a medium bowl, combine the tuna, olive oil, lemon juice, parsley, capers, red pepper flakes, oregano, and black pepper. Toss to coat.

Place the greens on a large plate and spoon the tuna salad on top. Top with the artichoke hearts, tomato wedges, cucumber, and sun-dried tomatoes.

Note: The tuna salad itself can be prepared ahead of time and stored in the refrigerator for easy, grab-and-go lunches throughout the week. If you want to prep the other ingredients ahead, store them in separate containers so that the greens don't wilt.

CHICKEN, APPLE, AND ALMOND SALAD

If you make my Emergency Roast Chicken (page 64), as I do about once a week, you'll inevitably find yourself with leftovers. As you very well know, reheating roasted chicken the next day, especially the white meat, is a fool's errand—it comes out dry and chewy. Instead of nuking your leftovers in the microwave, try making this delicious chicken, apple, and almond salad. It's quick, easy, and versatile.

I usually make a double batch and pack it in individual servings, alongside some leafy greens, for grab-and-go breakfasts and lunches. If you're living your post-Whole30 Food Freedom, try it between a couple slices of your favorite bread, gluten-free or otherwise!

In a large bowl, toss together all the ingredients. Taste and season with salt and pepper as needed. Cover and refrigerate until ready to serve. The salad will keep in the refrigerator for up to 5 days.

2 cups diced leftover roasted chicken

2 celery stalks, thinly sliced

½ shallot, finely chopped

½ Granny Smith apple, peeled, cored, and diced

3 tablespoons 30-Mississippi Mayonnaise (page 230)

1 tablespoon whole-grain or Dijon mustard

2 tablespoons unsalted dry-roasted almonds

1 tablespoon sherry vinegar

Kosher salt and freshly ground black pepper

Gluten-Free

Dairy-Free

Whole30

Paleo

Grain-Free

Time: 15 minutes

CARROT AND GARLIC SALAD

Gluten-Free

Dairy-Free

Whole30

Keto-Friendly

Paleo

Grain-Free

Time: 10 minutes, plus 30 minutes of marinating

2 pounds carrots, grated

¼ cup 30-Mississippi Mayonnaise (page 230)

2 garlic cloves, finely chopped

½ teaspoon kosher salt

Walk into any Russian delicatessen worth its salt and there will be at least thirty different cold salads in the glass display case. Chances are, a carrot and garlic salad like this will be one of them. It's commonly made with raisins and sometimes walnuts, but my parents never added either of those when I was growing up, so this pared-down version is what I've come to like best.

In a large bowl, toss together all the ingredients until well combined. Cover and refrigerate for at least 30 minutes before serving.

ASIAN BROCCOLI SALAD WITH CRISPY SHALLOTS

This Asian broccoli salad ideally should be prepared at least 1 hour before serving so that the flavors can develop; it can also be prepared the day before and refrigerated overnight. The crispy shallots, however, should be made shortly before serving so that they don't go soggy. And take care—the shallots can burn before you know it and will continue to brown after you remove them from the heat, so be sure to keep an eye on them and adjust the heat accordingly as they cook.

In a large bowl, whisk together the mayonnaise, vinegar, coconut aminos, sesame oil, garlic, and ginger until smooth. Add the broccoli, onion, and carrots and toss to coat. Cover with plastic wrap and refrigerate for at least 1 hour and up to overnight.

When ready to serve the salad, in a small, nonstick skillet, combine the avocado oil and shallot and cook over medium-low heat, stirring frequently, until the shallot is golden brown and crispy, about 15 minutes. Transfer the crispy shallots to a plate lined with a paper towel to drain excess oil.

Transfer the broccoli salad to a large serving platter. Garnish with the crispy shallots and sesame seeds.

½ cup 30-Mississippi Mayonnaise (page 230)

2 tablespoons rice vinegar

2 tablespoons coconut aminos

1 tablespoon toasted sesame oil

3 garlic cloves, finely grated

1 teaspoon finely grated fresh ginger

2 heads broccoli, cut into 2-inch florets

½ cup finely diced red onion

½ cup shredded carrots

1 tablespoon avocado oil

1 large shallot, thinly sliced

1 tablespoon sesame seeds, for garnish

Gluten-Free

Dairy-Free

Whole30

Keto-Friendly

Paleo

Grain-Free

Sugar-Free

Time: 20 minutes, plus at least 1 hour of marinating

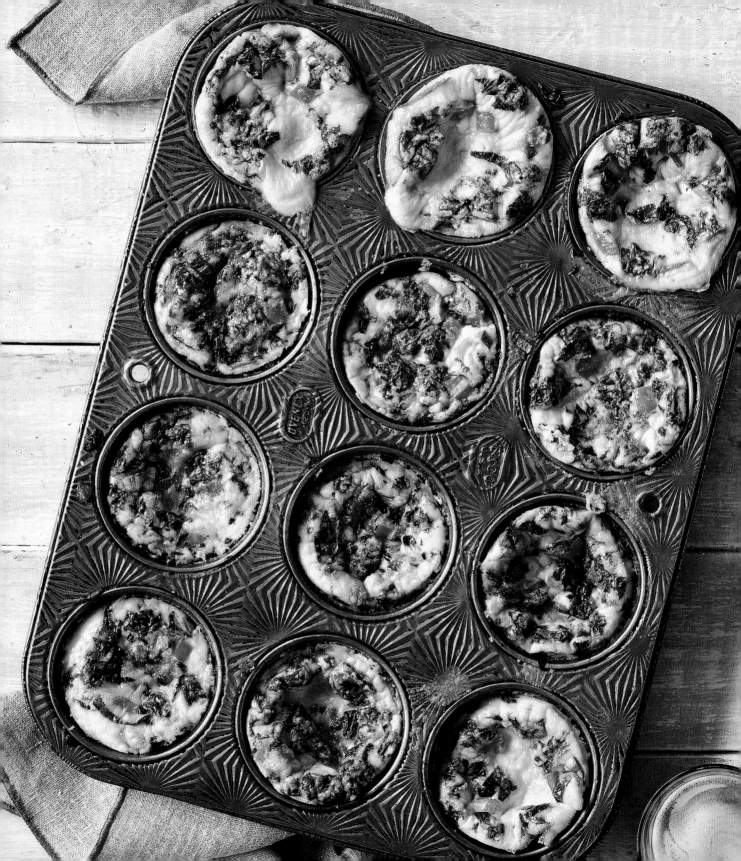

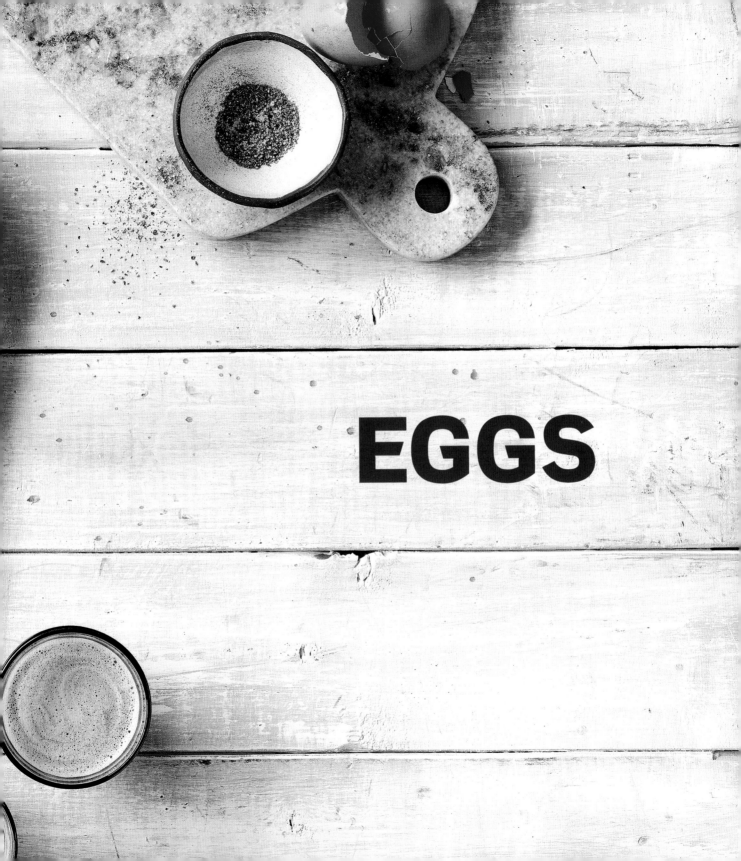

EGGS

CLASSIC DEVILED EGGS

Gluten-Free

Dairy-Free

Whole30

Keto-Friendly

Paleo

Grain-Free

Sugar-Free

Time: 30 minutes

12 large eggs

½ cup 30-Mississippi Mayonnaise (page 230)

1½ tablespoons Dijon mustard

Kosher salt

¼ cup capers packed in brine, drained, for garnish

¼ cup loosely packed fresh dill, finely chopped

1 teaspoon smoked paprika, for garnish

There are few things I love seeing at a party more than a great DJ and some deviled eggs. This classic appetizer has stood the test of time and continues to deliver as one of my all-time favorite things to make and eat. For the prettiest presentation, you'll need to use a piping bag fitted with a wide star tip. If that's too much to ask—and if it is, I understand—then simply use a zip-top plastic bag with one of the corners cut off instead.

Fill a large bowl with ice and water and set it nearby.

Bring a large pot of water to a boil over high heat. Using a slotted spoon, slowly lower the eggs into the water, being careful not to crack them on the bottom of the pot. Cook the eggs for exactly 12 minutes for hard yolks and whites. Transfer the eggs to the ice bath and let cool for at least 5 minutes.

Peel the eggs and slice them in half lengthwise. Gently separate the yolks from the whites and place them in separate medium bowls. Set the whites aside.

Transfer the yolks from the bowl to a fine-mesh strainer and use a spoon to gently push them through back into the bowl. Add the mayonnaise and mustard, season with salt, and mix until completely smooth.

Arrange the egg whites cut-side up on a platter. Transfer the yolk mixture to a piping bag fitted with a wide star tip and pipe about 1 tablespoon of the mixture into each of the egg whites. (If you don't have a piping bag, transfer the yolk mixture to a zip-top plastic bag and cut a small bit of one corner off.)

Garnish the deviled eggs with the capers and dill. Dust each with a pinch of the paprika and serve.

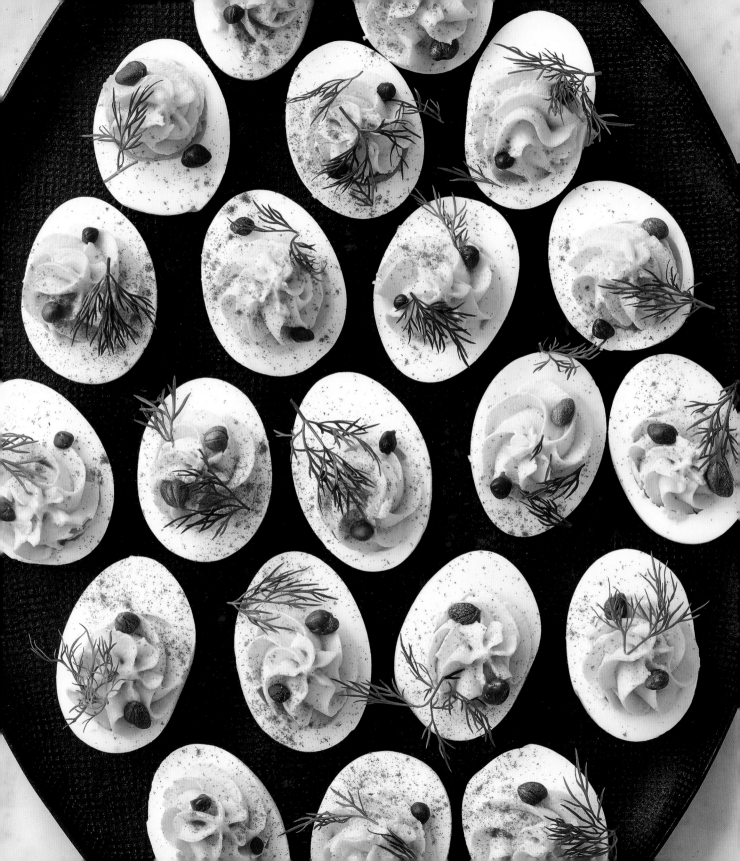

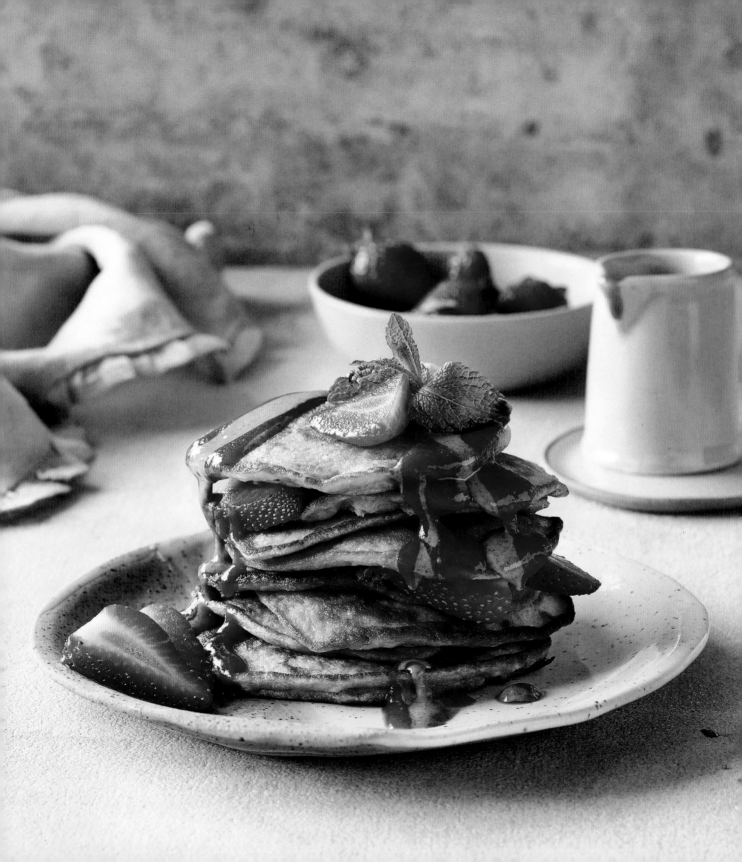

MARCELA'S PALEO PANCAKES WITH STRAWBERRY COULIS

I still remember the day my sister-in-law, Marcela, came over to show me this easy Paleo pancake recipe. My mind was blown, not only because there were so few ingredients, but also because the texture and taste were so much better than any of the other Paleo pancakes I had tried. Most Paleo pancakes are made with a combination of almond flour and coconut flour, both of which are dense and gritty, and tend to result in pancakes that crumble around the edges. Marcela's pancakes were crispy on the outside with light, spongy centers. They're the closest thing I've had to my mother's *oladi* (a type of Russian silver-dollar pancake made with kefir), and I've been addicted to them ever since.

Here I take the pancakes to the next level by drizzling them with almond butter and a simple strawberry coulis. It sounds fancy, but it really couldn't be easier.

MAKE THE STRAWBERRY COULIS: In a 2-quart saucepan, combine the strawberries, lemon juice, and honey (if using). Bring to a simmer over medium-high heat and cook until the strawberries have thawed and softened, 10 to 15 minutes. Remove the pot from the heat and use an immersion blender to puree the strawberries until smooth. (Alternatively, let the strawberries cool, then transfer to a blender and puree.) For a smoother sauce, pass the coulis through a fine-mesh strainer.

For the Strawberry Coulis:

2 cups frozen strawberries

1 tablespoon fresh lemon juice

1 tablespoon honey, agave nectar, or pure maple syrup (optional)

For the Pancakes:

4 large ripe bananas

4 large eggs

½ cup plus 2 tablespoons tapioca starch or cassava flour

3 tablespoons coconut oil, plus more if needed

For Serving:

¼ cup almond butter, room temperature

8 fresh mint leaves, for garnish (optional)

Gluten-Free
Dairy-Free
Paleo
Grain-Free

Time: 30 minutes

recipe continues

MAKE THE PANCAKES: In a medium bowl, mash the bananas with a fork until smooth. Add the eggs and whisk to combine. Whisk in the tapioca starch until smooth.

In a large nonstick skillet, melt the coconut oil over medium-low heat. Spoon in the batter to form silver-dollar-size pancakes and cook until the pancakes are golden brown on both sides and the edges are crispy, 2 to 3 minutes per side. Transfer the pancakes to a plate and repeat with the remaining batter, adding more coconut oil between batches, if needed.

TO SERVE: Arrange the pancakes on four individual plates and drizzle them with the strawberry coulis and the almond butter. Garnish with the mint leaves, if desired.

EGG SALAD
WITH DILL

My mom made this egg salad for us growing up. It's delicious, quick, and easy, and can be made ahead of time for grab-and-go breakfasts. You can spoon it over a bed of leafy greens or into lettuce cups, or, for an epic breakfast slider, sandwich it between two Twice-Fried Plantains (page 218).

Fill a large bowl with ice and water and set it nearby.

Bring a large pot of water to a boil over high heat. Using a slotted spoon, slowly lower the eggs into the water, being careful not to crack them on the bottom of the pot. Cook the eggs for exactly 12 minutes for hard yolks and whites. Transfer the eggs to the ice bath and let cool for at least 5 minutes.

Peel the eggs. Using a cheese grater, grate each egg into a medium bowl. (Alternatively, you can push them through the holes of a wire rack to quickly "chop" them.)

Add the mayonnaise, onion, dill, and salt. Stir to thoroughly combine. Taste and adjust the salt as desired. Serve, or cover and store in the refrigerator for up to 5 days.

10 large eggs

⅔ cup 30-Mississippi Mayonnaise (page 230)

½ cup finely chopped Vidalia onion

½ cup finely chopped fresh dill

½ teaspoon kosher salt, plus more as needed

Gluten-Free

Dairy-Free

Whole30

Keto-Friendly

Paleo

Grain-Free

Sugar-Free

Time: 35 minutes

SMOKED SALMON SCRAMBLE WITH CHIVES

Gluten-Free

Dairy-Free

Whole30

Keto-Friendly

Paleo

Grain-Free

Sugar-Free

Time: 15 minutes

8 large eggs

2 tablespoons ghee or grass-fed butter

4 ounces no-sugar-added smoked salmon, thinly sliced into ribbons

2 tablespoons finely chopped fresh chives

Freshly ground black pepper

Next to a perfectly cooked French omelet, soft-scrambled is my favorite way to enjoy eggs. For a special treat, I like to stir through ribbons of smoked salmon. The smoked fish is packed with flavor, healthy fat, and protein.

Unlike the rubbery, chewy scrambled eggs you might find at an all-you-can-eat hotel breakfast bar, these soft-scrambled eggs are delicate and moist. There are three helpful tips when it comes to perfect soft-scrambled eggs:

1. Use a smaller skillet than you think you'll need. Reducing the surface area safeguards against the eggs drying out as you drag them across the pan (see tip #2).
2. Gently drag the eggs from the outer edges of the pan toward the center rather than trying to break them apart with your spatula. This results in a fluffier texture.
3. Transfer the eggs to a plate just before they've finished cooking in the pan and let the residual heat do the rest of the work.

The flavor of smoked salmon intensifies as it cooks, so the trick here is to fold it into the eggs just before serving them. This way, they are evenly scattered throughout without overpowering the eggs.

In a medium bowl, whisk the eggs vigorously until smooth.

In an 8-inch nonstick skillet, melt the ghee over medium-low heat, about 1 minute. Pour in the eggs and, using a spatula, gently drag the eggs from the outer edges of the pan toward the center. Cook, repeating this motion, until the eggs are only slightly runny, about 2 minutes. Add the salmon and cook, continuing to drag the eggs toward the center, until the eggs are cooked to the desired consistency, about 1 minute more.

Garnish with the chives, season with pepper, and serve immediately.

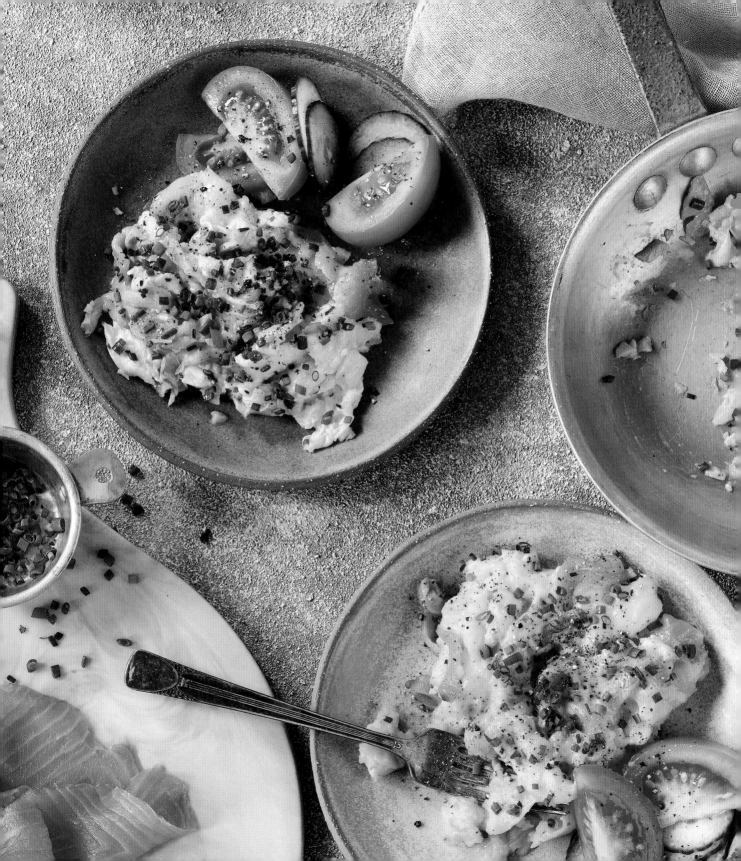

SABICH PLATTER

Gluten-Free
Dairy-Free
Whole30
Paleo
Grain-Free
Sugar-Free

Time: 70 minutes

For the Fried Eggplant:

1 large Italian eggplant

Kosher salt

¼ cup extra-virgin olive oil

⅓ cup arrowroot starch

For Serving:

2 tablespoons amba (mango sauce)

2 cups Chopped Salad (page 6)

4 hard-boiled eggs, peeled and thinly sliced

¼ cup Tahini Sauce (page 240)

2 tablespoons Zhug (page 246)

1 tablespoon unsalted sunflower seeds, toasted, for serving

Sabich is a wildly popular Israeli street food that was first introduced by Iraqi immigrants in the 1950s. It usually consists of a warm pita stuffed with slices of perfectly fried eggplant, sliced hard-boiled egg, chopped salad, tahini, sometimes hummus, usually Zhug (page 246), and almost always *amba* (pureed, quick-pickled mango). Amba can be purchased at most Middle Eastern grocers and even at Trader Joe's. Just be sure to check the ingredients list—there should be no artificial sweeteners, fillers, or preservatives.

Though *sabich* refers to the combination of these ingredients, in my mind, the eggplant is the star of the show. It makes or breaks the dish, which is why I spent the better part of a week slicing, frying, and eating my weight in eggplant while testing this recipe.

Here are my major takeaways:

1. Slice the eggplant as evenly as possible. Since you'll be shallow frying it in a very small amount of oil, you want to achieve the most contact with the oil as possible. Any undulation in the eggplant slice will cause it to cook unevenly, albeit slightly. It's not a deal breaker, but it's worth striving for a perfect slice.

2. Salt and drain the eggplant for at least 30 minutes. Lightly rubbing a small amount of kosher salt on each side of the eggplant slices will help draw out their bitter liquid, which will otherwise permeate your sabich. Resting the salted eggplant slices between paper towels proved to be the most effective method; the absorbent fibers help pull out the liquid. (Another popular option for draining eggplant is resting the slices on a wire rack, but since the metal is reactive, it can actually impart bitterness, not draw it out, undoing all your hard work!)

3. Dredge the sliced eggplant in arrowroot starch. After you've drained the eggplant, give them a light dusting of the starch. Not only does the starch make for a crispy and delicious finished product, it helps prevent the eggplant from absorbing too much oil as

recipe continues

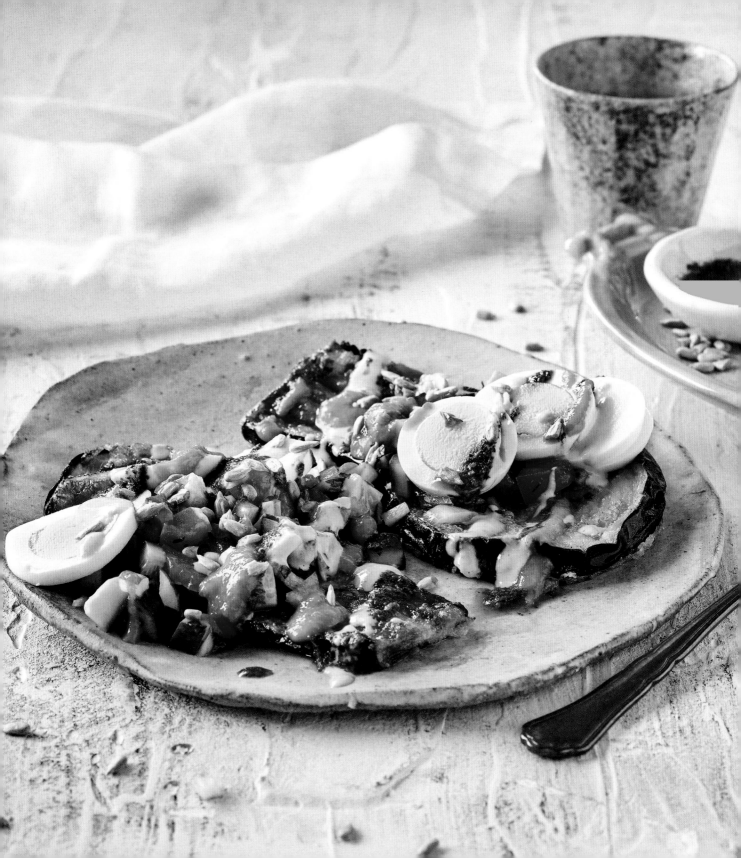

it fries. I also strongly urge you to only dredge the eggplant in the arrowroot starch immediately before frying. Otherwise, the arrowroot will turn gummy. When testing this recipe without arrowroot starch, I found that two slices of eggplant absorbed as much as ¼ cup of oil, versus significantly less with the starch. I also tested cassava flour and tapioca starch, both of which resulted in inferior flavor.

4. Pat the fried eggplant with paper towels after frying. I like to gently pat each fried slice with a clean paper towel after it comes out of the hot oil. This will absorb excess oil and prevent the eggplant from tasting greasy.

5. Serve immediately. You can absolutely prepare all the other ingredients for your sabich the day before. You can also definitely slice and salt the eggplant ahead of time, up to 3 to 4 hours. However, as mentioned, you do NOT want to dredge or fry the eggplant until immediately before serving. The beauty of this recipe is just how crispy and crunchy the eggplant gets from that light dusting of arrowroot starch.

MAKE THE FRIED EGGPLANT: Line a baking sheet with paper towels.

Trim the top of the eggplant and discard. Cut the eggplant lengthwise into ½-inch-thick slices, making them as flat as possible so that they fry evenly. Season both sides of each eggplant slice with salt. Arrange the slices in a single layer on the lined baking sheet. Top with another layer of paper towels and press down on the eggplant. Let the eggplant sit for 30 to 45 minutes to drain.

In a large nonstick skillet or sauté pan, heat the olive oil over medium-high heat until glistening. Line a second baking sheet with paper towels and set it nearby.

Put the arrowroot starch on a baking sheet or in a deep bowl. Pat the eggplant slices dry with a paper towel and lightly dredge them in the arrowroot starch to coat both sides.

Carefully transfer the eggplant to the hot oil and cook until golden brown on the bottom, 4 to 5 minutes. Flip and cook until the eggplant is golden brown on the second side, crispy, and tender, 3 to 4 minutes. Transfer the eggplant to the paper towels and gently pat them with another paper towel to absorb excess oil.

TO SERVE: In a small bowl, stir together the amba and 2 tablespoons water until smooth.

Divide the eggplant slices between two plates. Top with the chopped salad, followed by two eggs each. Drizzle with the tahini sauce, zhug, and amba. Sprinkle the sunflower seeds over the top and serve.

FLORENTINE EGG CUPS

Gluten-Free

Dairy-Free

Whole30

Keto-Friendly

Paleo

Grain-Free

Sugar-Free

Time: 40 minutes

1 tablespoon ghee, plus more for greasing

1 shallot, finely chopped

½ red bell pepper, diced

Kosher salt and freshly ground black pepper

3 cups loosely packed baby spinach, finely chopped

11 large eggs

½ cup full-fat coconut milk

4 ounces no-sugar-added smoked salmon, thinly sliced into ribbons

Breakfast always seems to be the most challenging meal for me. I don't have much time or appetite in the morning, so prepping something the day before always helps. Egg cups are a great option for batch cooking breakfast ahead of time. They can be eaten cold or reheated in the toaster oven or microwave. Enjoy them on their own or with your favorite hot sauce, salsa, or guacamole.

Preheat the oven to 325°F. Grease a 12-cup muffin tin with ghee and set it on a rimmed baking sheet to catch any spills.

In a large nonstick skillet, melt the ghee over medium heat. Add the shallot and bell pepper, season with a pinch each of salt and black pepper, and cook, stirring, until the vegetables are slightly softened, about 3 minutes. Add the spinach and cook, stirring, until wilted, about 2 minutes. Taste and adjust the salt and pepper as desired. Remove the pan from the heat.

In a large bowl, whisk together the eggs and coconut milk until thoroughly combined and smooth.

Using a spoon, distribute the vegetable mixture evenly among the prepared muffin cups. Divide the sliced salmon evenly over the vegetables, then ladle the egg mixture over the top. Bake until a toothpick or cake tester inserted into the center of an egg cup comes out clean, about 25 minutes.

Serve immediately, or let cool, transfer to an airtight container, and store in the refrigerator for up to 4 days.

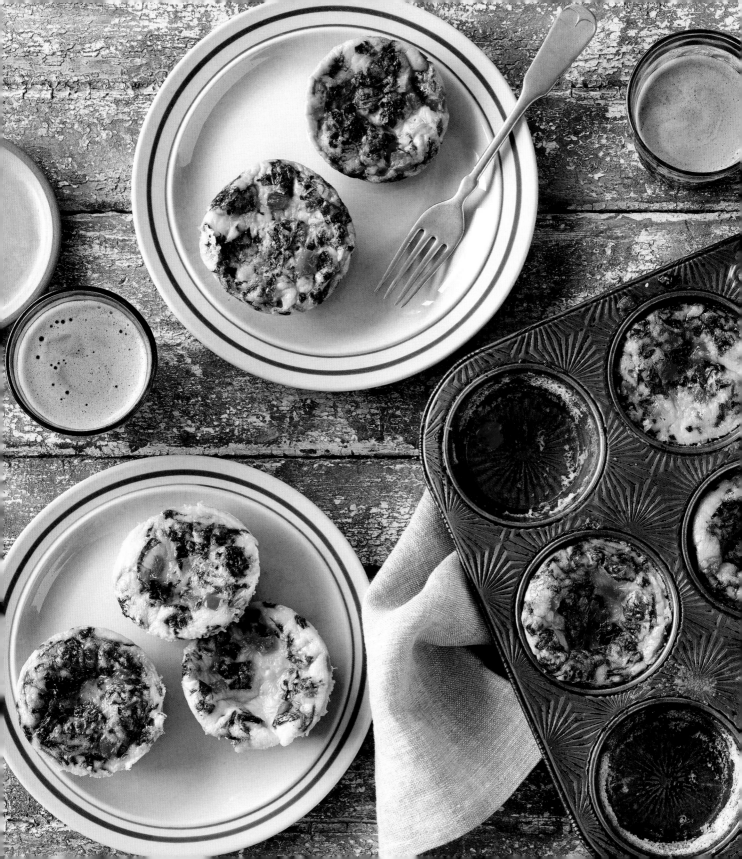

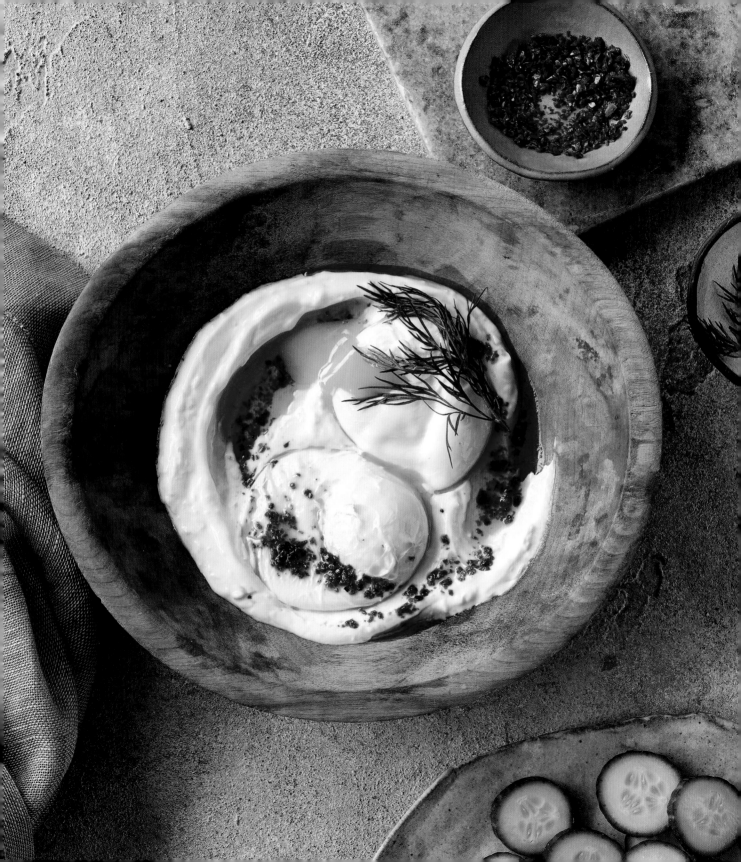

TURKISH POACHED EGGS WITH COCONUT YOGURT AND ALEPPO-SPICED GHEE

I've never been to Turkey, but it's on my list of top places to visit, not least because of the amazing food! *Cilbir*, made with poached eggs, garlicky yogurt, and a chile-infused butter, is just one of the delicacies I'd love to try. Just like sabich (page 28), it's one of those odd combinations that works! Sourcing dried Turkish chiles, such as Aleppo or Urfa pepper, might be your biggest hurdle, but it's worth the effort. Look for a local Middle Eastern grocer first. If that fails, order the ingredients online. If that doesn't work, use your favorite ground chile.

As with my Civilake Tizaki (page 236), I play with tradition here by using a dairy-free "fauxgurt" made from coconut milk. If you're not a fan of coconut flavor in general, feel free to use any dairy-free yogurt you prefer. I also replace conventional butter with ghee, a clarified butter that is virtually dairy-free. The result is a very tasty, if untraditional, take on a Turkish-inspired breakfast. This is typically enjoyed with freshly baked bread, but roasted potatoes make a nice substitute for soaking up the yogurt and runny egg yolks. Try it with a side salad or raw veggies for a well-rounded breakfast.

¼ cup ghee

1 teaspoon Aleppo pepper

1 cup coconut "fauxgurt" (see Civilake Tizaki (Coconut Tzatziki), page 236)

1 garlic clove, finely chopped

4 large eggs

½ cup torn fresh dill, for garnish

Gluten-Free

Dairy-Free

Whole30

Keto-Friendly

Paleo

Grain-Free

Sugar-Free

Time: 15 minutes

In a small saucepan, stir together the ghee and Aleppo pepper. Melt the ghee over medium-low heat, about 3 minutes. Reduce the heat to its lowest setting to keep the mixture warm until ready to serve.

In a small bowl, whisk together the "fauxgurt" and garlic. Set aside.

Bring a medium saucepan of water to a very gentle simmer, around 185°F, over medium heat.

recipe continues

Crack an egg into a fine-mesh strainer set over a bowl and give it a swirl to separate any of the scraggly whites. Using a large spoon, swirl the water in the pot to create a vortex. While the water is swirling, carefully add the egg. Repeat this process with each egg until they are all in the pot. Cook until the egg whites are firm and the yolks are still soft, 4 to 5 minutes. Stir the water occasionally to keep the eggs from coming in contact with the bottom of the pot.

Using a slotted spoon, carefully remove each egg from the water and transfer 2 eggs to each serving bowl, making sure not to puncture the yolks. Spoon the garlicky "fauxgurt" over the top of the eggs and drizzle with the Aleppo-spiced ghee. Garnish with the dill and serve immediately.

KALE STEM FRITTATA

If you make my Kale and Walnut Pesto (page 238), you might be left scratching your head thinking about what to do with all of the leftover kale stems. Whatever you do, don't toss them out! They're perfectly edible and high in fiber. Instead, try adding them to a frittata the following morning. They're fairly neutral in flavor and quite filling. Just be sure to finely chop and sauté them first so that they soften. Otherwise, they can be a bit stringy.

The beauty of a frittata is that you can incorporate just about any fillings you like or have on hand. This version keeps things simple with a bit of crispy bacon, shallot, red bell pepper, and fresh tomato to finish.

Preheat the oven to 325°F.

Place the bacon slices in a 10-inch oven-safe nonstick or cast-iron skillet and set it over medium heat. Cook, turning the bacon once or twice, until golden brown and slightly crispy, about 6 minutes. Transfer to paper towels to drain excess grease and set aside. Pour off all but 2 tablespoons of the rendered bacon fat in the skillet.

In a medium bowl, whisk together the eggs and coconut milk until thoroughly combined and smooth. Set aside.

Return the skillet to medium heat, add the kale stems, and season with salt and black pepper. Cook, stirring, until slightly softened, 3 to 4 minutes. Add the bell pepper and shallot and cook, stirring, for 2 minutes more, until softened. Pour the egg mixture into the pan and add the bacon. Gently stir to evenly distribute the ingredients.

Top with the tomato slices and transfer the pan to the oven. Cook for 20 to 25 minutes, until a toothpick or cake tester inserted into the center comes out clean. Serve immediately.

4 slices bacon, thinly sliced

8 large eggs

¼ cup full-fat coconut milk

¼ cup finely chopped kale stems

Kosher salt and freshly ground black pepper

½ red bell pepper, diced

1 shallot, diced

1 large Roma (plum) tomato, thinly sliced

Gluten-Free

Dairy-Free

Whole30

Keto-Friendly

Paleo

Grain-Free

Sugar-Free

Time: 45 minutes

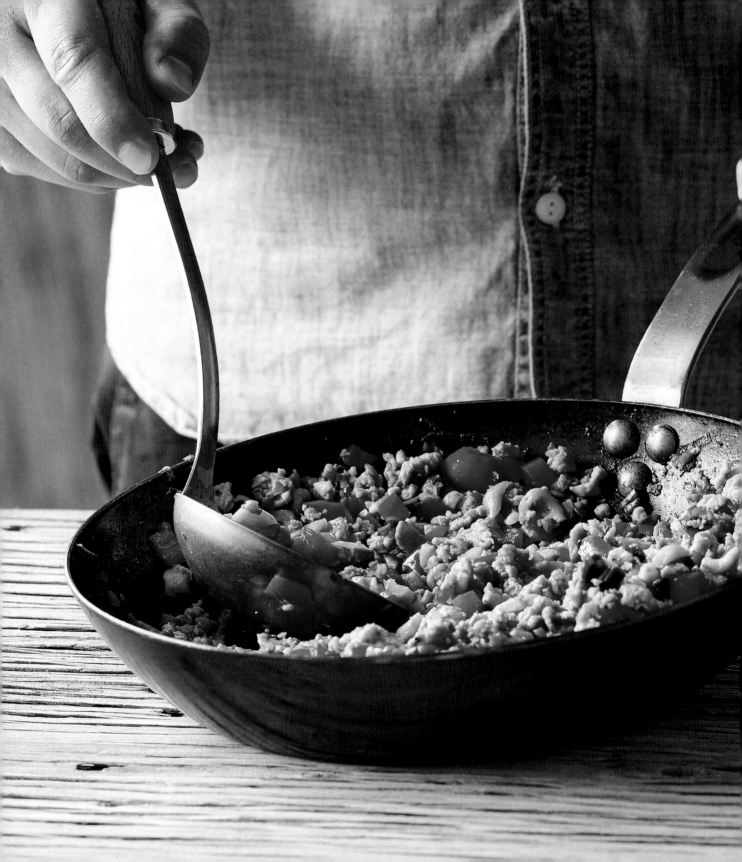

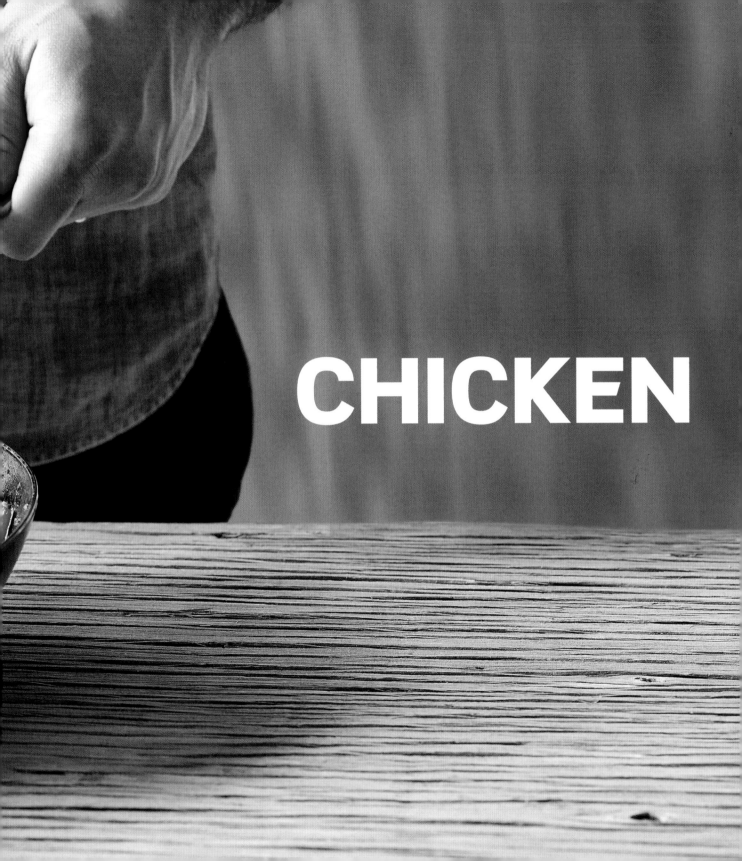

CHICKEN

CHICKEN SCHNITZEL

Gluten-Free

Dairy-Free

Paleo

Grain-Free

Sugar-Free

Time: 30 minutes

2 (6-ounce) boneless, skinless chicken breasts

¼ cup arrowroot starch

¼ cup cassava flour

2 large eggs

¼ teaspoon kosher salt

⅛ teaspoon freshly ground black pepper

3 tablespoons avocado oil

1 teaspoon sesame seeds, for serving

Flaky sea salt, for serving

Cassava flour is a fantastic (though harder to find) alternative flour and is both gluten-free and has a low glycemic index. I particularly like cassava flour for schnitzel because of its coarser grind, which gets nice and crispy. Be sure to first dust the chicken in some arrowroot starch. This acts as a binder for the egg wash, which, in turn, helps the cassava flour stick.

Try serving the schnitzel with my Creamy Fennel and Celery Slaw (page 5), Oven Fries (page 200), or with a side of Whole30 Tartar Sauce (page 245).

Line a baking sheet with a wire rack.

Set the chicken breasts on a cutting board. Place one hand flat on one chicken breast and extend your fingers away from the board for safety. With your knife blade held parallel to the cutting board, slice the chicken breast in half horizontally. Repeat with the second chicken breast. Lay the chicken slices flat on the cutting board, cover them with plastic wrap, and pound them with a meat mallet or rolling pin until they are approximately ¼ inch thick.

Place the arrowroot starch, cassava flour, and eggs into three separate bowls. Season the cassava flour with the salt and pepper. Add 2 tablespoons water to the eggs and whisk vigorously until frothy.

Dredge each piece of chicken in the arrowroot starch to coat both sides, then dip into the egg wash, letting any excess drip off. Dredge in the seasoned cassava flour to coat and set aside on a large plate.

In a large nonstick skillet, heat the avocado oil over medium-high heat for 1 to 2 minutes, until it shimmers. Carefully add the breaded chicken to the hot oil and cook until golden brown, about 4 minutes. Flip and cook for 2 minutes more, until browned on the second side. Transfer the cooked schnitzel to the wire rack. Sprinkle them evenly with the sesame seeds and season each with a tiny pinch of flaky sea salt. Serve immediately.

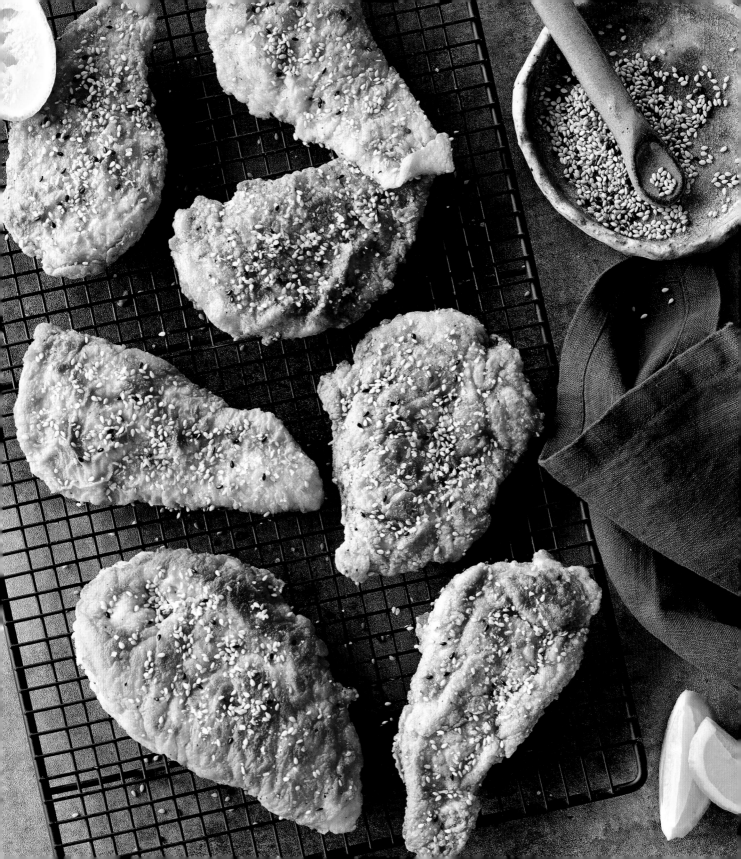

CHICKEN MEATBALLS
WITH SUN-DRIED TOMATO CREAM SAUCE

Gluten-Free

Dairy-Free

Whole30

Keto-Friendly

Paleo

Grain-Free

Sugar-Free

Time: 40 minutes

For the Meatballs:

2 pounds ground chicken

1 large egg

¼ cup finely chopped fresh parsley leaves

2 tablespoons finely chopped sun-dried tomatoes packed in olive oil, drained

1 shallot, finely chopped

2 garlic cloves, finely chopped

2 teaspoons kosher salt

1 teaspoon dried basil

½ teaspoon freshly ground black pepper

2 tablespoons extra-virgin olive oil, plus more as needed

One of the most popular recipes on CookPrimalGourmet.com is my Sun-Dried Tomato Chicken Burger. It's super easy to prepare, and the flavors scream "summertime," especially when topped with a garlicky basil aioli. Here I transform the burgers into meatballs and serve them in a quick-and-easy sun-dried tomato cream sauce. The sauce uses virtually the same ingredients as the meatballs, which amplifies all the flavors.

The best part is, this recipe comes together in a single pan and takes less than 30 minutes to prepare! Try serving the meatballs over a bed of mashed potatoes or cauliflower "grits" (see Adobo Shrimp with Cauliflower "Grits" and Collard Greens, page 162).

MAKE THE MEATBALLS: In a large bowl, combine the ground chicken, egg, parsley, sun-dried tomatoes, shallot, garlic, salt, basil, and pepper. Mix with your hands until well combined. Rub a small amount of olive oil on your hands and form the mixture into meatballs slightly larger than golf balls, setting them on a baking sheet as you roll them.

In a large sauté pan, heat the olive oil over medium-high heat. Add the meatballs to the pan and cook until browned on all sides and cooked through, about 15 minutes. Transfer the meatballs to a platter and set aside.

MAKE THE SUN-DRIED TOMATO CREAM SAUCE: Wipe the sauté pan clean with a paper towel, return the pan to medium-high heat, and pour in the olive oil. Add the bell pepper and shallot and cook, stirring, until slightly softened, 3 to 4 minutes. Add the garlic and cook, stirring, for 30 seconds. Add the coconut milk, sun-dried tomatoes, and mustard and season with salt and black pepper. Cook, stirring occasionally, until the sauce has reduced by at least a quarter, about 4 minutes. Taste and adjust the seasoning, if desired.

Remove the pan from the heat, add the meatballs to the sauce, and toss to coat. Let the meatballs sit until they have warmed through, about 3 minutes. Serve immediately.

For the Sun-Dried Tomato Cream Sauce:

1 tablespoon extra-virgin olive oil

1 red bell pepper, diced

1 shallot, finely chopped

2 garlic cloves, finely chopped

1¼ cups full-fat coconut milk

2 tablespoons coarsely chopped sun-dried tomatoes packed in olive oil, drained

1 tablespoon Dijon mustard

Kosher salt and freshly ground black pepper

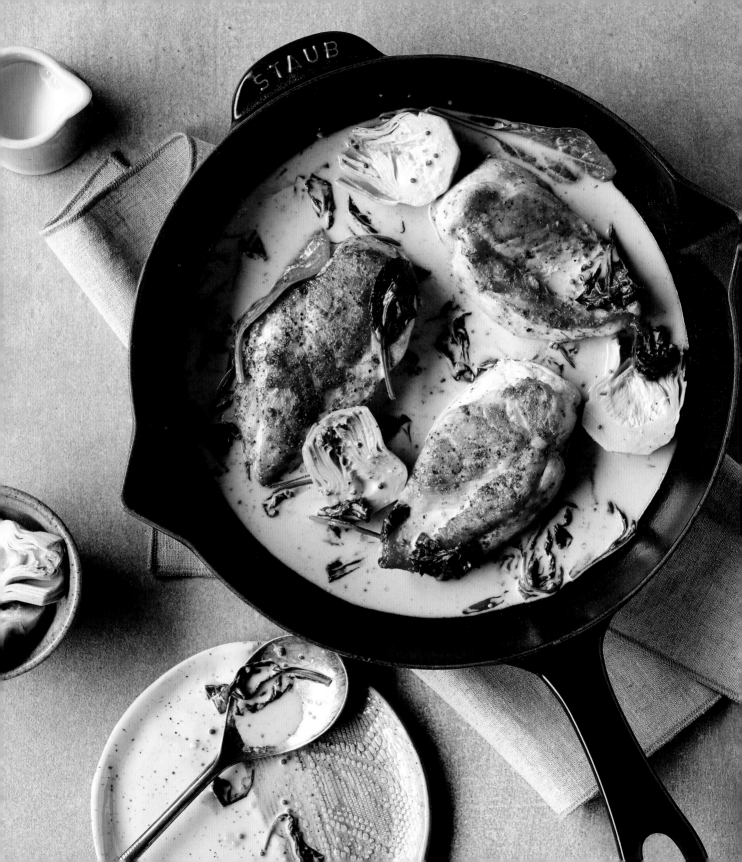

CHICKEN WITH SPINACH AND ARTICHOKE CREAM SAUCE

If I'm at a restaurant and there's a spinach and artichoke dip on a menu, I'm ordering it. I just can't resist. This is a lighter and healthier riff on the classic appetizer, one of my favorites. Rather than enjoy it as a dip, I make it into a meal by pairing it with some pan-seared chicken breasts and serving it over mashed potatoes or cauliflower grits (see page 162) to soak up all the sauce. It takes under 20 minutes from start to finish and is every bit as rich, creamy, and delicious as the original, minus all the dairy!

Set the chicken breasts on a cutting board. Place one hand flat on one chicken breast and extend your fingers away from the board for safety. With your knife blade held parallel to the cutting board, slice the chicken breast in half horizontally. Repeat with the remaining chicken breasts. Pat the chicken slices dry with paper towels and season both sides with salt and pepper.

In a large skillet, heat the olive oil over medium-high heat. Add the chicken and cook until golden brown on both sides and cooked through, 4 to 5 minutes per side. Transfer the chicken to a plate and set aside.

Add the garlic to the skillet and cook, stirring continuously, for 30 seconds. Add the stock and cook, scraping up any browned bits from the bottom of the pan with your spoon, for 1 to 2 minutes. Add the coconut milk, ¼ teaspoon salt, and ¼ teaspoon pepper and cook until the sauce has reduced by half, 3 to 4 minutes. Stir in the mustard.

Add the spinach and artichokes and cook until the spinach has wilted, about 2 minutes. Taste and season with salt and pepper as desired. Return the chicken to the pan and serve immediately.

4 (6-ounce) boneless, skinless chicken breasts

Kosher salt and freshly ground black pepper

2 tablespoons extra-virgin olive oil

2 garlic cloves, finely chopped

½ cup chicken stock

1 cup full-fat coconut milk

1 tablespoon Dijon mustard

⅓ cup loosely packed baby spinach

1 (14-ounce) can artichoke hearts packed in water, drained and sliced in half

Gluten-Free
Dairy-Free
Whole30
Keto-Friendly
Paleo
Grain-Free
Sugar-Free

Time: 30 minutes

Note: Feel free to substitute chicken thighs for a slightly richer-tasting finished product.

MOJO LOCO CHICKEN WINGS

Gluten-Free

Dairy-Free

Whole30

Paleo

Grain-Free

Sugar-Free

Time: 40 minutes, plus 4 hours of marinating

½ cup fresh orange juice

¼ cup fresh lime juice

¼ cup extra-virgin olive oil

4 garlic cloves, peeled

1 jalapeño

1 teaspoon dried oregano

1 tablespoon ground coriander

3½ to 4 pounds chicken wings

Kosher salt and freshly ground black pepper

¼ cup loosely packed fresh cilantro leaves

8 fresh mint leaves

Mojo (pronounced *mo-ho*) is a delicious marinade found throughout South America and the Caribbean. It's commonly made with a combination of bitter orange (*naranja agria*), garlic, and oregano. The variations, however, are endless. In some countries, mint is added; in others, bay leaf. In nearly all cases, it's delicious, and makes a versatile marinade that can be used on pork (see page 150), chicken, beef, and even seafood. Here the *mojo* does double duty, first as a marinade for the chicken wings and then as a spicy sauce, to which I add fresh cilantro and mint for a boost of flavor and color.

In a blender, combine the orange juice, lime juice, olive oil, garlic, jalapeño, oregano, and coriander. Blend on high speed until smooth.

Season both sides of the chicken wings with 3 teaspoons salt and ½ teaspoon pepper. Place the wings in a large zip-top plastic bag and pour in half the marinade. Massage the wings to coat with the marinade, then squeeze out as much air from the bag as possible and seal the bag. Set it on a rimmed baking sheet and refrigerate for at least 4 hours or up to overnight.

Add the cilantro and mint to the remaining marinade and blend until smooth. Taste and season with salt and pepper as desired. Transfer the mojo sauce to a jar, cover, and refrigerate until needed.

Position an oven rack in the lower third of the oven and preheat the oven to 425°F. Line a rimmed baking sheet with parchment paper.

Arrange the wings in a single layer on the prepared baking sheet (discard the marinade left in the bag) and roast for 30 to 35 minutes, until the wings are golden brown and register 165°F on an instant-read thermometer.

Serve the wings with the mojo sauce alongside for dipping.

Notes: If you can find bitter orange juice, use it. As a substitute here, I've used two parts fresh orange juice to one part fresh lime juice.

This mojo has a bit of kick to it, hence the "Loco" in the title. For a milder version, remove the seeds from the jalapeño before adding it to the marinade.

As I mention in the recipe for my Ragin' Cajun Wings (page 51), I don't bother flipping the wings halfway through the cooking time. Instead, I prefer to let the oven do all the work.

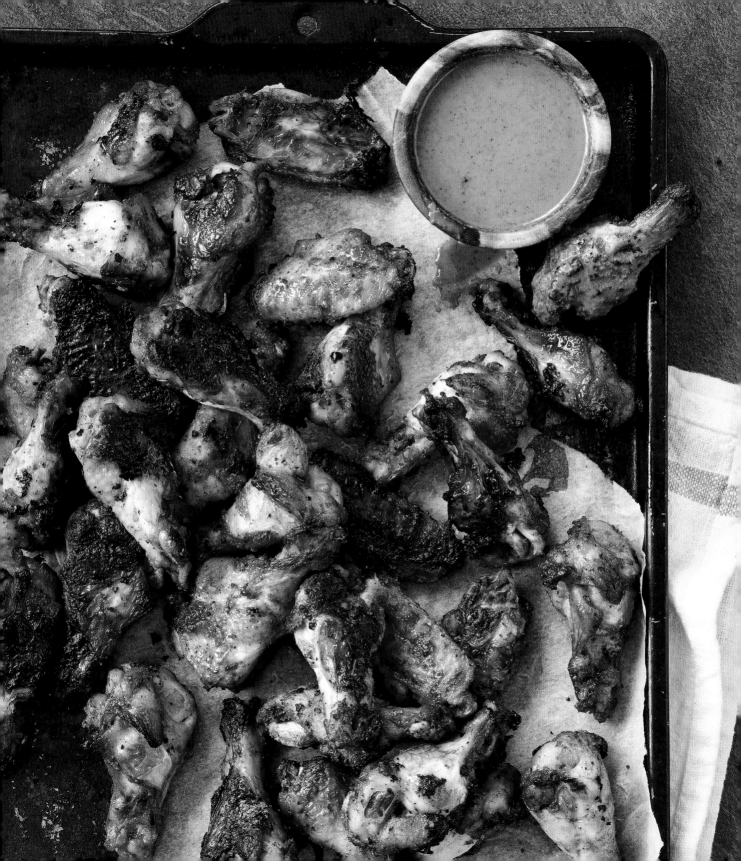

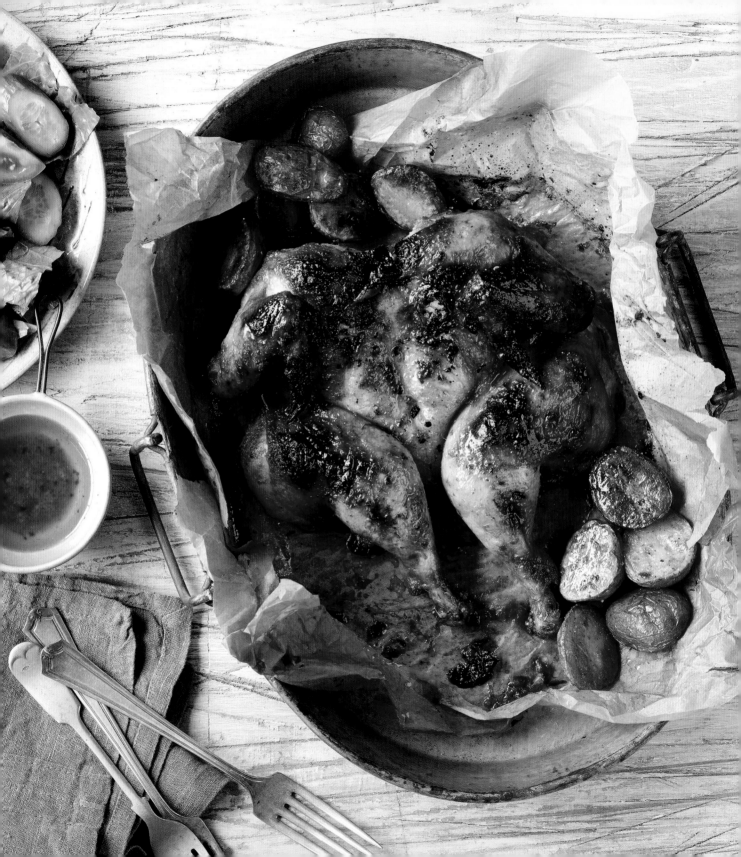

PIRI PIRI CHICKEN

A staple menu item at Portuguese *churrasquerias*, piri piri chicken (also called pili pili or peri peri) derives its name from the peppers traditionally used in the dish's marinade. Piri piri peppers arrived in Portugal by way of southeastern Africa and thereafter became popularized by the charred rotisserie chickens that came to bear their name. Though it's very easy to find piri piri condiments and marinades in major grocery stores, most of them are filled with sugars, fillers, and other weird ingredients. Less easily found are the piri piri peppers themselves. Instead, I use red finger chiles for their color, fruitiness, and mild heat. If they're unavailable, you can substitute Anaheim peppers. For an added kick, I also add a pinch of cayenne, but you can omit this if you like things milder.

Spatchcocking the chicken (butterflying it by removing the backbone) will reduce the cooking time and expose more of the skin, giving it a chance to get crispy (for more on why I prefer this method, see Emergency Roast Chicken, page 64).

As far as pairings go, you can't beat some simple roast potatoes and a garden salad with piri piri chicken.

In a blender, combine the onion, olive oil, vinegar, lemon juice, garlic, chiles, ginger, salt, smoked paprika, sweet paprika, oregano, cayenne, and ¼ cup water. Blend on high speed until smooth.

Dry the chicken with paper towels. Using sharp kitchen shears or a sharp knife, cut along one side of the backbone, leaving the other side attached. Lay the chicken breast-side up on a cutting board and press down on the breastbone with your hands to flatten the chicken. Put the chicken in a large zip-top plastic bag and pour in the marinade. Massage the marinade all over the chicken, then squeeze as much air out of the bag as possible and seal. Place it on a baking sheet with the chicken breast-side down and refrigerate for at least 4 hours or up to overnight.

recipe continues

1 small yellow onion, halved

¼ cup extra-virgin olive oil

¼ cup red wine vinegar

Juice of ½ lemon

4 garlic cloves, peeled

2 fresh red finger chiles (or Anaheim chiles, if not available)

1 (1-inch) piece fresh ginger, peeled

1 tablespoon kosher salt

1 teaspoon smoked paprika

1 teaspoon sweet paprika

1 teaspoon dried oregano

½ teaspoon cayenne pepper, plus more if desired

1 (2½- to 3-pound) whole chicken

Gluten-Free

Dairy-Free

Whole30

Keto-Friendly

Paleo

Grain-Free

Sugar-Free

Time: 55 minutes, plus 4 hours of marinating

Preheat the oven to 425°F. Line a 4-inch-deep roasting pan with parchment paper.

Remove the chicken from the marinade, letting any excess drip off (discard the bag). Place the chicken in the prepared roasting pan and roast on the bottom rack for 40 to 45 minutes, until the thickest part of the thigh registers 165°F on an instant-read thermometer. Use a turkey baster or large spoon to baste the chicken with the rendered juices in the pan.

Set the oven to broil, but keep the chicken on the bottom rack (putting the parchment paper closer to the broiler could cause it to catch fire). Broil for 4 to 5 minutes, until the skin is golden brown and crispy.

Transfer the chicken to a grooved cutting board to catch any juices and let it rest for 5 to 10 minutes before carving and serving.

RAGIN' CAJUN WINGS

Put my Ragin' Cajun Spice Rub to good use with these chicken wings. They're super easy to make and can be easily adjusted to feed a game-day crowd. When I'm baking chicken wings, I don't bother flipping them halfway through. This is partly because I'm an inherently lazy human being, but mostly because you lose a lot of heat when you open the oven door. This is especially true of older ovens, which aren't as efficient as newer convection models. To ensure a crispy wing, I lay them flat on a rimmed baking sheet lined with parchment paper and make sure that there's a bit of space between each to maximize cooking surface area. I also bake them at a high temperature on the lowest rack of the oven, because that's where it's hottest. The result is a crispety, crunchety chicken wing that's also moist and juicy.

Preheat the oven to 425°F. Line a baking sheet with parchment paper.

Dry the chicken wings thoroughly with a paper towel. Place them in a large bowl, add the avocado oil, and toss to coat. Add the Cajun seasoning and toss to coat.

Arrange the wings in a single layer on the prepared baking sheet and bake on the bottom rack of the oven for 30 to 35 minutes, until the internal temperature registers 165°F on an instant-read thermometer and the wings are crispy. Serve immediately with the carrot and celery sticks.

2 pounds chicken wings

1 tablespoon avocado oil

2 tablespoons Ragin' Cajun Spice Rub (page 259)

2 large carrots, cut into large matchsticks, for serving

3 celery stalks, cut into large matchsticks, for serving

Gluten-Free

Dairy-Free

Whole30

Paleo

Grain-Free

Sugar-Free

Time: 40 minutes, plus 4 hours of marinating

CHICKEN SHAWARMA
WITH BOOTLEG GARLIC SAUCE

Gluten-Free

Dairy-Free

Whole30

Keto-Friendly

Paleo

Grain-Free

Sugar-Free

Time: 30 minutes

1½ pounds boneless, skinless chicken thighs (about 8)

3 tablespoons avocado oil

1 teaspoon granulated onion

1 teaspoon ground cumin

1 teaspoon ground coriander

1 teaspoon kosher salt

½ teaspoon ground turmeric

½ teaspoon cayenne pepper

½ teaspoon ground cinnamon

½ teaspoon ground cardamom

1 teaspoon ground sumac, for garnish

½ cup Bootleg Garlic Sauce (page 234), for serving

Chicken shawarma usually takes two days to prepare. The meat is marinated overnight before it is skewered on a very large metal spit and slowly roasted for hours. Before serving, shawarma is sliced by hand or with an electric meat shaver and is often crisped on a griddle. The whole process is time-consuming and requires specialty kitchen equipment, which makes it particularly difficult for home cooks who want to try their hand at preparing it.

This version, believe it or not, takes around 30 minutes to prepare and delivers comparable results. Purists may throw shade, but I would put it up against some of my favorite shawarma spots in Toronto—especially with some Bootleg Garlic Sauce drizzled on top. The secret to the chicken lies in the spice rub and cooking technique. I tinkered with this combination of spices for over a year before finally nailing it down. Yes, it's a long list, but I strongly encourage you to make it as directed before trying out any changes. Each spice brings something different to the table, and they work together beautifully. The same goes for the sumac, which I like to dust over the shawarma before serving.

As far as technique, slicing the chicken before cooking it is key. It increases the surface area of the meat available for spices to cling to and for the chicken to brown. Since you'll be cooking the chicken at high heat, it's important to use an oil with a high smoking point. Avocado oil works best because it can withstand higher temperatures and is neutral in flavor. Likewise, use a pan made from a material that is suitable for high-heat cooking, such as cast iron or carbon steel. This is particularly important because you have to cook the chicken without moving it for 6 to 8 minutes to develop a crust before flipping. A stainless-steel pan may work, but you run the risk of the meat sticking to the bottom, and a nonstick

recipe continues

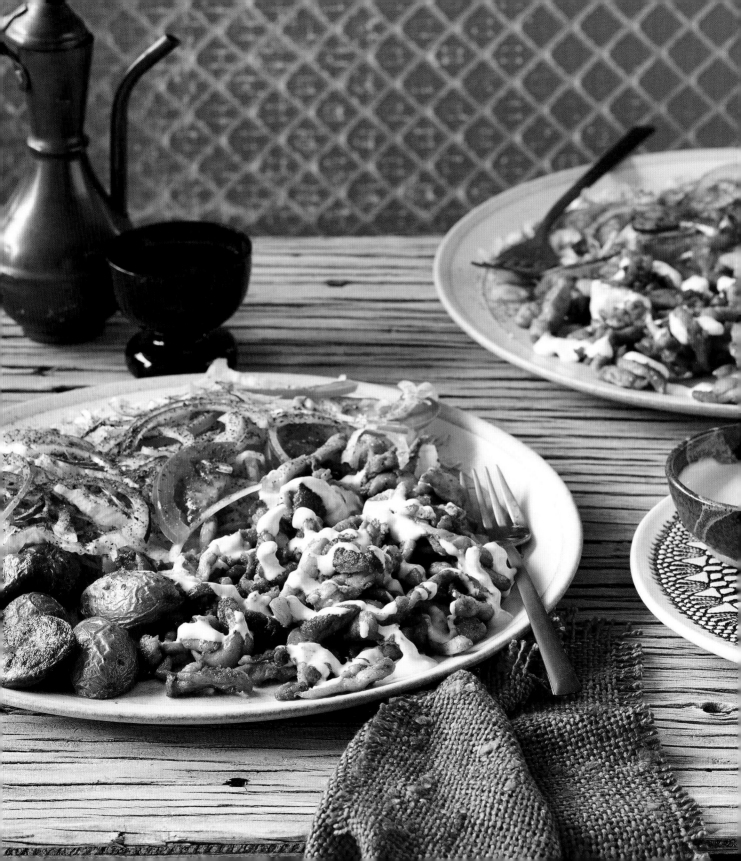

pan just won't develop a crispy enough crust (and that's aside from concerns about nonstick materials breaking down at higher temperatures).

Try serving the shawarma with roasted potatoes or Oven Fries (page 200), Fauxttoush (page 8), and some Bootleg Garlic Sauce or The Dracula Killer (Toum) (page 242).

Pat the chicken thighs dry with paper towels and slice them into roughly ⅛-inch-thick strips. Put the sliced chicken in a large bowl and add 2 tablespoons of the avocado oil, the granulated onion, cumin, coriander, salt, turmeric, cayenne, cinnamon, and cardamom. Toss to coat.

Heat a large cast-iron skillet over medium heat for 5 minutes. Add the remaining 1 tablespoon avocado oil and increase the heat to medium-high. Arrange the chicken in the pan in a single layer and cook, undisturbed, until browned on the bottom, 6 to 8 minutes. Flip the chicken and cook, stirring occasionally, until it is cooked through and crispy, 4 to 5 minutes.

Remove the pan from the heat and sprinkle the chicken with the sumac. Serve immediately with the garlic sauce.

JERK CHICKEN

I've eaten my fair share of jerk chicken over the years. With so many Jamaican and Caribbean restaurants in Toronto and the GTA (Greater Toronto Area), it's kind of hard not to. But I really have to thank my big brother, Julian, for my mild obsession with everything jerk. He's always had a knack for seeking out hidden gems all over the city and then convincing me to go to these places with him to eat. To be fair, it was never that hard to get me to go.

I'm certainly no expert, but I wouldn't hesitate to put this homemade version up against some of the best I've had. It's spicy, but not painfully so, very flavorful thanks to a very easy Jerk Rub (page 257), and it always comes out incredibly juicy. It also happens to be Paleo-friendly and Whole30-compliant, but you'd never guess it.

For best results, let the chicken marinate overnight. The apple cider vinegar will help tenderize the meat and the flavors will penetrate down to the bone. Personally, I'm a dark-meat kind of guy, but you could just as easily use chicken breast here. If so, I recommend going with bone-in, skin-on pieces for maximum flavor.

In the warmer months, head outside and try grilling the jerk chicken! Start by cooking it over indirect heat for about 30 minutes before searing it over direct heat to finish. Just keep an eye on it, because the spices in the rub can easily scorch if left unattended. Note that cooking times will vary depending on the efficiency of your oven or the heat of your grill, if you're going that route.

For pairings, you'd be hard-pressed to find better sides than my Caraway Cabbage Coleslaw (page 2) and some Sweet Plantains (Maduros) (page 210).

8 chicken quarters

Kosher salt

1 cup Jerk Rub
(page 257)

Gluten-Free
Dairy-Free
Whole30
Paleo
Grain-Free
Sugar-Free

Time: 50 minutes, plus at least 4 hours of marinating

Liberally season both sides of the chicken quarters with salt and place them in a large zip-top plastic bag. Add the jerk rub to the bag. Massage to coat the chicken with the rub, then squeeze as much air out of the bag as possible and seal. Place it on a rimmed baking sheet and refrigerate for at least 4 hours or up to 24 hours.

recipe continues

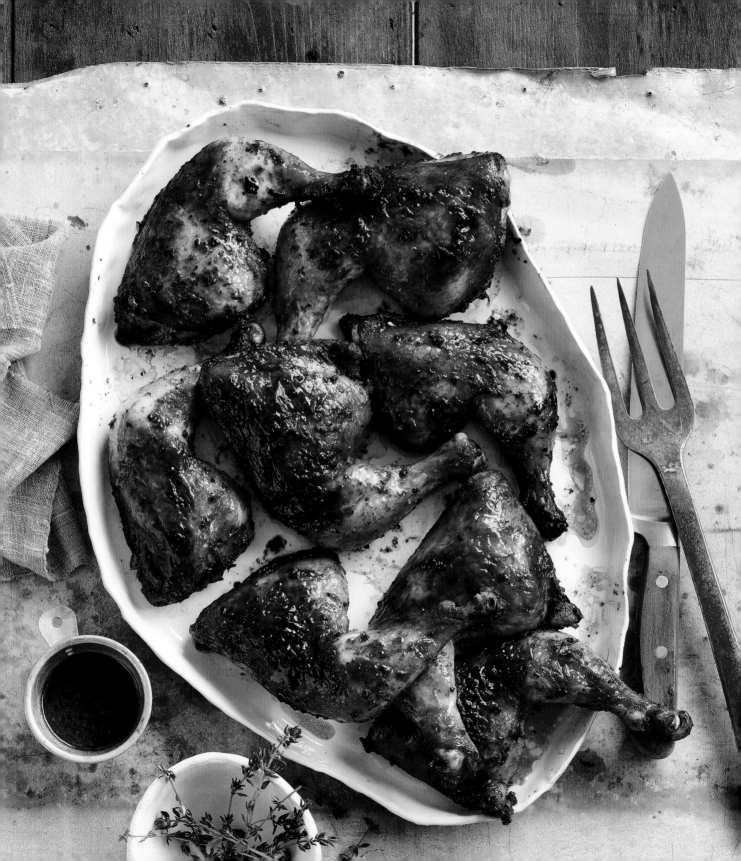

Preheat the oven to 425°F. Line a rimmed baking sheet with parchment paper.

Remove the chicken from the bag, letting any excess rub drip off (discard the bag). Place the chicken skin-side up on the prepared baking sheet and roast on the bottom rack for 35 to 40 minutes, until the thickest part of the thigh registers 165°F on an instant-read thermometer. Check the chicken halfway through the cooking time; if you notice it is browning unevenly, rotate the baking sheet 180 degrees.

Let the chicken rest in the pan for 5 minutes before serving.

KUNG PAO LETTUCE CUPS

Gluten-Free

Dairy-Free

Whole30

Keto-Friendly

Paleo

Grain-Free

Sugar-Free

Time: 25 minutes

2 tablespoons avocado oil

1 pound ground chicken

1 red bell pepper, diced

4 scallions, white and green parts separated and thinly sliced

¼ cup raw cashews

1 recipe Teriyaki Sauce (page 241)

Kosher salt

8 iceberg lettuce leaves, for serving

Iceberg lettuce is my preferred vessel here. It's crisp and holds up well as you handle the little bundles of delicious, saucy chicken. Boston or butter lettuce is also a good option because of the size and shape of its leaves, but it lacks crunch. Then again, you can just as easily serve this as a main course over some Cauliflower Rice (page 205) or steamed rice, if you're living your Food Freedom. I'll let you decide how to eat them. You're the boss, applesauce.

Heat a large cast-iron or carbon-steel wok or skillet over medium heat for 5 minutes. Increase the heat to high and pour in the avocado oil. Heat until shimmering, then add the ground chicken. Cook, stirring and breaking up the meat as it cooks, until the chicken is browned and all the moisture has evaporated, 4 to 5 minutes. Add the bell pepper, the scallion whites, and the cashews and cook, stirring, until the peppers have softened slightly, 2 to 3 minutes. Stir in the teriyaki sauce and toss to coat. Cook, stirring occasionally, until the sauce has reduced by about one-quarter, 2 to 3 minutes.

Sprinkle in the scallion greens and stir. Taste and season with salt as desired.

Transfer the chicken to a serving bowl and serve with the iceberg lettuce leaves on a plate alongside.

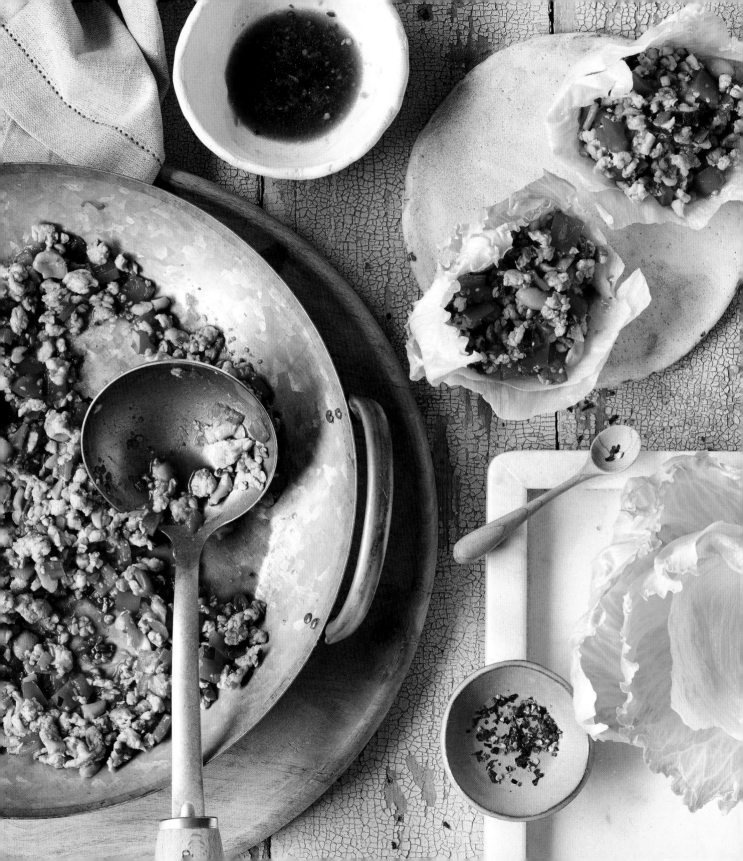

CHICKEN BONE BROTH

Gluten-Free

Dairy-Free

Whole30

Keto-Friendly

Paleo

Grain-Free

Sugar-Free

Time: 3 hours
to 24 hours,
depending on
method

Pressure cooker
method: 3 hours
and 15 minutes

Slow cooker
method:
24 hours

Stovetop method:
24 hours

1½ to 2 pounds
assorted chicken
bones, raw or
previously roasted

2 carrots, cut in half

2 celery stalks,
cut in half

1 onion, cut in half

1 chayote squash,
cut in half

1 large or 2 small
parsnips, cut in half

1 head garlic,
bottom trimmed and
discarded

½ cup loosely packed
fresh parsley

1 (2-inch) piece
fresh ginger

3 bay leaves

1 tablespoon apple
cider vinegar
(optional)

1 tablespoon
kosher salt

1 teaspoon whole
black peppercorns

Chicken bone broth is virtually identical to conventional chicken stock, but differs in its cooking time: whereas chicken stock can be prepared in about an hour (see page 71), bone broth is often cooked for up to 72 hours. The extended cooking time is necessary to extract the collagen and other nutrients from the bones. If your bone broth solidifies like gelatin when you refrigerate it, that's a good indication that you cooked it right.

Bone broth is believed to improve the health and quality of your skin, repair torn cartilage and damaged joints, heal leaky gut syndrome, build stronger teeth, and boost your immune system—basically, it's great for your overall health. It can be enjoyed by the cup or used to make soups, stews, and sauces. It can be prepared in a stockpot on the stovetop, in a slow cooker, or in a pressure cooker (electronic or stovetop). Any way you cook it, the goal is the same: to extract the collagen and other nutrients from the bones.

There are a few ways to maximize the amount of collagen you're getting in your bone broth. Some people swear by adding a tablespoon of apple cider vinegar, which is believed to help break down the bones and extract collagen. Personally, I don't find this to be all that effective, and it adds a slightly sour note to my broths. I've had much more success with including parts of the chicken that are rich in collagen to begin with, such as feet, thighs, legs, and backbones. I also find that it helps significantly to cook the broth low and slow for as long as possible, upward of 48 hours in a slow cooker, for example.

As far as cooking methods go, each one has its pros and cons. I've taken the liberty of providing each one here so that you can experiment and see which you like best. Personally, I prefer the taste of broths made using the stovetop and slow cooker methods. As the liquid evaporates, the broth reduces and its flavors concentrate. The downside is the length of time it takes to cook.

Pressure cooking, on the other hand, can save you as much as 21 hours! But the flavor is a bit different. I also find that the silicone gasket on electronic pressure cookers ends up smelling like old gym clothes after you've made several batches of bone broth. So if you notice some funk in your cuppa broth, it might be time to replace the gasket.

Regardless of which method you use, I recommend two things:

1.   Parboil the bones and skim off any foam that rises to the surface of the water. This will result in a less cloudy finished product.
2.   Make use of vegetable scraps in your bone broth. It's good to get into the habit of saving things like carrot skins, celery ends, and onion peels. Simply collect these scraps in a freezer-safe bag and store them in the freezer (do the same with any chicken bones and carcasses). Before long, you'll have enough aromatics to flavor your broth—not to mention reducing food waste and saving money.

PRESSURE COOKER METHOD: Put the chicken bones in a 6-quart pressure cooker and add water to cover. Set the pressure cooker to SAUTÉ and bring the water to a steady simmer. Cook, using a large spoon to skim off any foam that rises to the surface, for 10 to 12 minutes, or until the broth is no longer foaming.

Add the carrots, celery, onion, squash, parsnip, garlic, parsley, ginger, bay leaves, vinegar (if using), salt, peppercorns, and enough additional water to reach the max fill line. Cancel the SAUTÉ function and switch to MANUAL mode. Select HIGH pressure for 180 minutes (3 hours). Lock on the lid and set the valve to SEALING.

When the cooking time is up, allow the pressure to release naturally or quick-release it.

recipe continues

Set a fine-mesh sieve on top of a pitcher (I use my blender jar). Carefully pour the broth through the sieve and discard the solids. Let the broth cool.

SLOW COOKER METHOD: Put the bones in a 6-quart stockpot and add water to cover. Bring to a boil over high heat, reduce the heat to maintain a steady simmer, and cook, using a spoon to skim off any foam that rises to the surface, for 10 to 12 minutes, or until the broth is no longer foaming.

Transfer the bones and water to a 6-quart slow cooker. Add the carrots, celery, onion, squash, parsnip, garlic, parsley, ginger, bay leaves, vinegar (if using), salt, peppercorns, and enough additional water to reach the max fill line. Cover and cook on Low for 24 hours, or until you can easily crumble one of the chicken bones between your fingers.

Set a fine-mesh sieve on top of a pitcher (I use my blender jar). Carefully pour the broth through the sieve and discard the solids. Let the broth cool.

STOVETOP METHOD: Put the bones in a 5½-quart stockpot and add water to cover. Bring to a boil over high heat, reduce the heat to maintain a steady simmer, and cook, using a spoon to skim off any foam that rises to the surface, for 10 to 12 minutes, or until the broth is no longer foaming.

Add the carrots, celery, onion, squash, parsnip, garlic, parsley, ginger, bay leaves, vinegar (if using), salt, peppercorns, and enough additional water to fill to about 1 inch below the top of the pot. Cover the pot and cook on the lowest possible heat for 24 hours, or until you can easily crumble one of the chicken bones between your fingers.

Set a fine-mesh sieve on top of a pitcher (I use my blender jar). Carefully pour the broth through the sieve and discard the solids. Let the broth cool.

TO STORE: Pour the cooled broth into room-temperature or warm mason jars. If you'll be freezing the broth, be sure to leave 1½ to 2 inches of headroom to prevent the jars from bursting (the broth will expand as it freezes). Alternatively, freeze the broth in large silicone ice molds; once the broth has frozen, transfer the ice cubes to a freezer-safe bag for easy storage. The broth will keep in the refrigerator for up to 1 week or in the freezer for up to 6 months.

EMERGENCY ROAST CHICKEN

Gluten-Free

Dairy-Free

Whole30

Keto-Friendly

Paleo

Grain-Free

Sugar-Free

Time: 60 minutes

1 (2½ to 3-pound) whole chicken

1 tablespoon coarsely chopped fresh rosemary

Kosher salt and freshly ground black pepper

One of the most popular recipes on CookPrimalGourmet.com is my Emergency Roast Chicken, and for good reason. It's dead simple to make, has only two ingredients (not including salt and pepper), and cooks in 45 minutes. It always comes out with perfectly crispy skin and juicy meat. And when paired with a recipe from the Salads chapter (see page 1) or the Vegetables chapter (see page 185), it's a great back-pocket weeknight meal.

As far as technique goes, you can't go wrong with spatchcocking. It is by far my preferred way to prep a chicken for roasting. The bird cooks evenly and looks beautiful on the table. To spatchcock a chicken, cut along the backbone with a pair of sharp kitchen shears or a sharp knife so you can lay the whole bird out flat. Most people cut along both sides of the backbone and completely remove it, but I actually like to leave it attached on one side. This provides additional fat to render, which you can use to baste the bird before broiling. After all, this recipe doesn't call for any added oil. The meat and skin along the spine are also incredibly delicious when roasted, and nothing goes to waste this way! If you do insist on fully removing the backbone, put it in a zip-top freezer bag and freeze it to use for Mama's Chicken Soup (page 71) or Chicken Bone Broth (page 60).

Preheat the oven to 425°F. Line a 4-inch-deep roasting pan with parchment paper.

Pat the chicken very dry with paper towels. Using sharp kitchen shears or a sharp knife, cut along one side of the backbone, leaving the other side attached. Lay the chicken breast-side up on a cutting board and press down on the breastbone with your hands to flatten the chicken. Liberally season the chicken all over with the rosemary and salt and pepper. Transfer the chicken breast-side up to the prepared roasting pan.

Roast on the bottom rack of the oven for 40 to 45 minutes, until the thickest part of the thigh registers 165°F on an instant-read thermometer. Use a turkey baster or large spoon to baste the chicken with the juices from the pan.

Set the oven to broil, but keep the chicken on the bottom rack (putting the parchment paper closer to the broiler could cause it to catch fire). Broil for 4 to 5 minutes, until the skin is golden brown and crispy.

Transfer the chicken to a grooved cutting board to catch any juices and let it rest for 5 to 10 minutes before carving and serving.

WHOLE30 FAUXSOLE VERDE CON POLLO

Gluten-Free

Dairy-Free

Whole30

Keto-Friendly

Grain-Free

Sugar-Free

Time: 1 hour

For the Salsa Verde:

1½ pounds tomatillos, husked and washed well

1 jalapeño

1 poblano pepper

1 cubanelle pepper

¼ cup loosely packed fresh cilantro leaves

2 tablespoons fresh lime juice

1 teaspoon ground cumin

1 teaspoon ground coriander

Kosher salt, to taste

For the Soup:

2 tablespoons extra-virgin olive oil

1 yellow onion, diced

5 or 6 garlic cloves, smashed and peeled

Kosher salt

1½ pounds boneless, skinless chicken thighs (about 8)

3 white or yellow potatoes, peeled and cut into ¼-inch cubes

2 avocados, diced, for serving

Traditional Mexican posole derives its name from the hominy (*posole* in Spanish) used to make it. Although delicious, hominy is made from corn kernels, which are neither Paleo nor Whole30-compliant. Here I replace the hominy with diced, peeled yellow potatoes to make a "fauxsole." The potato gives the dish a similar appearance and imparts some texture. Before serving, I like to top the soup with thinly sliced red onion, fresh cilantro, and diced avocado. It's also very popular to add some thinly sliced cabbage or iceberg lettuce. For an extra bit of crunch, try shallow-frying some Cassava Flour Tortillas (page 226) in avocado oil until golden brown, crushing them, and sprinkling them over the soup. If you're living your Food Freedom, a bit of crumbled cotija cheese will take this to a whole other level.

This recipe makes an easy homemade salsa verde and uses it in the broth for the soup, but you can substitute 16 ounces of your favorite Whole30-compliant, store-bought Mexican salsa verde.

MAKE THE SALSA VERDE: Preheat the oven to 450°F. Line a baking sheet with parchment paper.

Place the tomatillos stem-side down on the prepared baking sheet, then arrange the jalapeño, poblano, and cubanelle peppers on the baking sheet as well. Roast for 25 to 30 minutes, until the tomatillos and peppers are slightly charred and begin to release their juices. Let cool for at least 5 minutes, then peel, stem, and seed the peppers and transfer the flesh to a blender or food processor and add the tomatillos.

Add the cilantro, lime juice, cumin, coriander, and salt to the blender and blend until smooth. Taste and season with salt as

recipe and ingredients continue

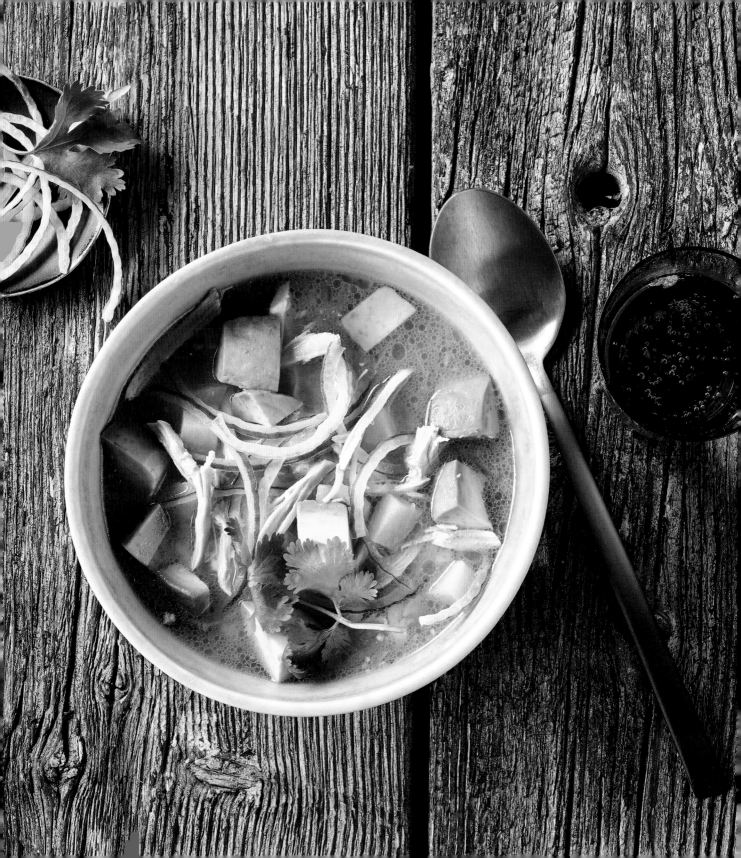

½ red onion, thinly
sliced, for serving

Fresh cilantro leaves,
for garnish

desired. Pour the salsa verde into a sealable container and set aside until ready to use. (The salsa will keep for up to 1 week in the refrigerator.)

MAKE THE SOUP: In a large Dutch oven or stockpot, heat the olive oil over medium heat. Add the onion, garlic, and a pinch of salt and cook, stirring occasionally, until the onion is soft and translucent, about 10 minutes. Add the chicken, potatoes, 2 cups of the salsa verde, and 10 cups of water to the pot. Bring to a low simmer and cook, skimming off and discarding any foam that rises to the surface, until the chicken registers 165°F on an instant-read thermometer at the thickest part of a thigh, 12 to 14 minutes.

Transfer the chicken to a bowl and let cool, then shred the meat with your hands or two forks. Return the shredded chicken to the pot and stir. Let the soup rest for 10 to 15 minutes before serving.

Ladle the soup into individual serving bowls. Garnish with the avocado, red onion, and cilantro. Store any leftover salsa in the refrigerator or reserve for another use.

MAMA'S ROAST CHICKEN WITH MONTREAL STEAK SPICE

Growing up, my mother would roast a chicken at least once a week. During the rest of the week, we were likely eating her chicken soup (see page 71). We ate chicken so often that at one point, I started protesting white meat, begging and pleading for everything from pizza pockets to cheeseburgers to grilled cheese sandwiches instead. I would bargain with promises of doing my homework early, mowing the lawn, shoveling snow off the driveway, or any number of other chores I despised. Realizing my mother wasn't going to budge and give in to my requests, I would dig deep and promise that I would get along with my brother for an entire week if she would just feed me some junk food! She rarely caved. The irony is that I now not only love roast chicken, I associate the smell of it with home and feelings of comfort and nostalgia. I never thought I'd see the day!

My mother's favorite way to roast chicken was to season the bird with Montreal steak spice. It wasn't until my early twenties that I realized just how delicious this chicken is, and it brings me great joy to share the recipe with you here. Naturally, I use a homemade Montreal steak spice in place of the store-bought stuff. It's lower in sodium and doesn't have any unnecessary refined vegetable oils in it.

1 (2½- to 3-pound) whole chicken

2 tablespoons extra-virgin olive oil or ghee

2 tablespoons Montreal Steak Spice (page 258)

Gluten-Free

Dairy-Free

Whole30

Keto-Friendly

Paleo

Grain-Free

Sugar-Free

Time: 60 minutes

Position a rack in the bottom third of the oven and preheat the oven to 400°F.

Pat the chicken very dry with paper towels and place it breast-side up on a rimmed baking sheet or in a roasting pan. Rub the chicken with the olive oil and season it with the Montreal steak spice. Roast on the bottom rack until the thickest part of the thigh registers 165°F

recipe continues

on an instant-read thermometer, 40 to 50 minutes. Baste the chicken with the rendered juices from the pan.

Set the oven to broil, but keep the chicken on the bottom rack (putting the parchment paper closer to the broiler could cause it to catch fire). Broil for 3 to 4 minutes, until the skin is golden brown and crispy.

Transfer the chicken to a grooved cutting board to catch any juices and let it rest for 10 minutes before carving and serving.

MAMA'S CHICKEN SOUP

This is my mama's chicken soup. It is the best chicken soup in the entire world. This isn't up for debate. This is a fact. It is science. It is math (1 + 1 = Mama's Chicken Soup!). Are we clear? When I was growing up, my mother made this chicken soup (a.k.a. "Jewish penicillin") at least once a week. We ate it so often that at one point, I never wanted to see it again. In addition to meeting her weekly chicken soup quota, she also made it on every single holiday, Jewish or otherwise (and continues to do so today). I would know it was a holiday when I saw that she used the chicken soup as a base for her Matzo Ball Soup (page 77), something I will never get tired of!

The recipe I'm sharing is a codified version of something intangible. Chicken soup, my mama's included, is an organic, living thing. It changes a little bit every time and doesn't need to be made by following any specific measurements. Chicken soup is something you can feel your way through, and improvisation is a part of the process. It is the jazz of the culinary world.

Of course, this is not something that comes easily to everyone. It takes practice and a great deal of trial and error. I have probably tried to re-create my mama's chicken soup no less than two dozen times, and it still doesn't hold a candle to hers. What can I say? She has that touch! But that shouldn't stop anyone, myself included, from trying. I'm happy to say that with this recipe, you can come very close to tasting my childhood. But you might need a few pointers along the way:

STOCK VS. SOUP: This is, for all intents and purposes, a recipe for chicken soup and is intended to be enjoyed as soup. If you have leftover liquid, you can pour it through a fine-mesh sieve to discard any flecks in the stock and store it in mason jars to be frozen and used in other recipes that call for chicken broth or stock.

4 chicken quarters

4 large carrots, unpeeled

2 yellow onions, unpeeled, cut in half

2 celery stalks, cut in half

1 large parsnip, unpeeled, cut in half

1 chayote squash, cut in half

1 small bunch dill, plus more for garnish

1 (2-inch) piece fresh ginger

1 head garlic, bottom trimmed and discarded

3 bay leaves

2 tablespoons kosher salt, plus more if needed

1 teaspoon whole black peppercorns

Freshly ground black pepper

Gluten-Free

Dairy-Free

Whole30

Keto-Friendly

Paleo

Grain-Free

Sugar-Free

Time: 1½ hours

recipe continues

CHICKEN

Store-bought stock doesn't hold a candle to this stuff. Try using it to make any number of soups or pan sauces, such as the sauce for my Steak au Poivre (page 87).

RAW VS. ROASTED: You don't have to use raw chicken, especially if you plan on using this recipe to make chicken stock. You can just as easily substitute a roasted chicken carcass or bones, as you would if making bone broth (see page 60). Roasted bones have a concentrated flavor that gets released into the broth as it slowly cooks. Using leftover bones is also a great way to reduce waste! The downside, of course, is that you won't have any shreds of chicken meat in the soup.

FRESH VS. SCRAPS: Likewise, using whole, fresh, beautiful produce to make the stock isn't absolutely necessary. As mentioned in my bone broth recipe (page 60), save vegetable scraps from other recipes you make throughout the week and use them to make stock. I keep a "stock bag" in the freezer for precisely this purpose. I add to it every time I peel an onion or carrot, trim celery, or confront those tiny cloves of garlic that are impossible to peel. However, it is virtually impossible for me to quantify carrot trimmings and onion peels. It's also very hard for me to explain how to cook without a recipe. Therefore, I recommend sticking to the ingredients and measurements for your first few tries. This way, you have a reference point from which you can improvise for future batches.

USE KOSHER OR HALAL CHICKEN: If you're going to use raw chicken parts, such as legs and thighs or even an entire bird, you may want to consider using kosher or halal meat. Unlike nonreligious butchering practices, one of the requirements in both kosher and

recipe continues

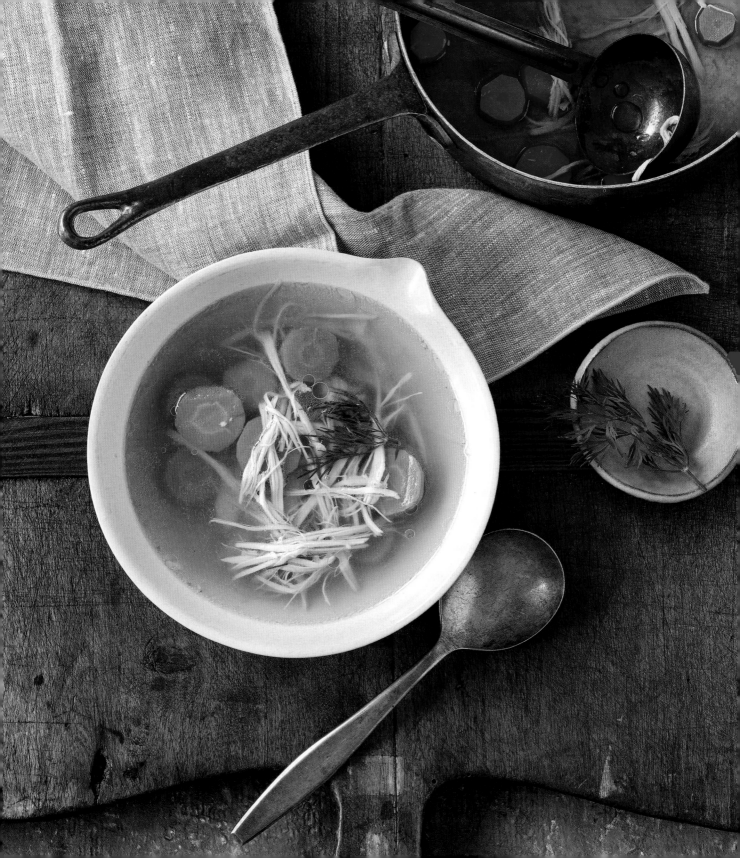

halal laws is for the blood to be drained from the animal. Religious considerations and debates aside, this will result in a less cloudy stock. Not to mention the fact that the animals must be slaughtered in a humane way, or the meat is considered inedible.

If, however, you are using the bones or carcass of a roasted bird, this is less of a concern, since most of the blood will have been cooked and/or drained after carving. On the other hand, many roasted chickens are first seasoned or marinated in any number of spices, etc., and these will inevitably color your stock. I once made stock from the remains of a batch of Ragin' Cajun Wings (page 51). While incredibly delicious, the stock was noticeably darker and redder than usual.

CLEAN VS. CLOUDY: When you do not skim the foam that rises to the surface of the liquid as you're cooking your stock, the stock will be cloudy. The foam is likely the result of solidified impurities in the meat. Over the years, I've become a bit of a stickler for clean and clear stocks. Although it's not the end of the world if I see some gray flecks floating around, I always strive for a less cloudy finished product by using the following techniques:

1) Simmer the chicken on its own in water for 10 minutes. Skim off any foam that rises to the surface before adding your vegetables and aromatics. This is the same technique I outline in my bone broth recipe (see page 60). One thing I've noticed is that while adding everything at once results in a more flavorful broth, the vegetables and herbs trap some of the foam and make it harder to skim off, so it can solidify later and linger in the stock.

2) Follow the recipe as outlined, but strain the cooked stock through a fine-mesh sieve or cheesecloth before serving. This will ensure maximum flavor and a clearer finished product.

KEEP THE SCHMALTZ: Although you should skim any foam that rises to the surface, you should definitely leave the fat globules. Those beautiful, shiny bubbles that dance across the surface of your soup are rendered chicken fat (a.k.a. schmaltz). This is the holy grail of Jewish delicacies and is pure, unadulterated flavor! You will notice significantly more schmaltz when using skin-on raw chicken, since most of the chicken fat is stored in the skin—making a case for using raw chicken as opposed to roasted bones.

In a 7½-quart stockpot or Dutch oven, combine the chicken, carrots, onions, celery, parsnip, squash, dill, ginger, garlic, bay leaves, salt, and peppercorns. Add enough water to fill the pot. Bring the water to a gentle simmer over medium heat. Cover and cook for 1¼ hours, using a spoon to skim off any foam that rises to the surface.

Remove the pot from the heat and use a large slotted spoon or spider to transfer the chicken to a bowl; let cool slightly. Discard all the vegetables except the carrots. Peel the carrots and slice them into 1-inch-thick discs. Set aside.

When the chicken is cool enough to handle, shred the meat with your hands or two forks. Discard the bones, skin, and cartilage. Return the shredded chicken to the pot along with the sliced carrots. Taste the soup and season with additional salt, if desired.

Ladle into individual bowls, garnish with dill and freshly ground black pepper, and serve.

Note: All of the vegetables are edible, and you can enjoy them in your soup, if you like. Personally, I am not a fan of the texture, so I discard them.

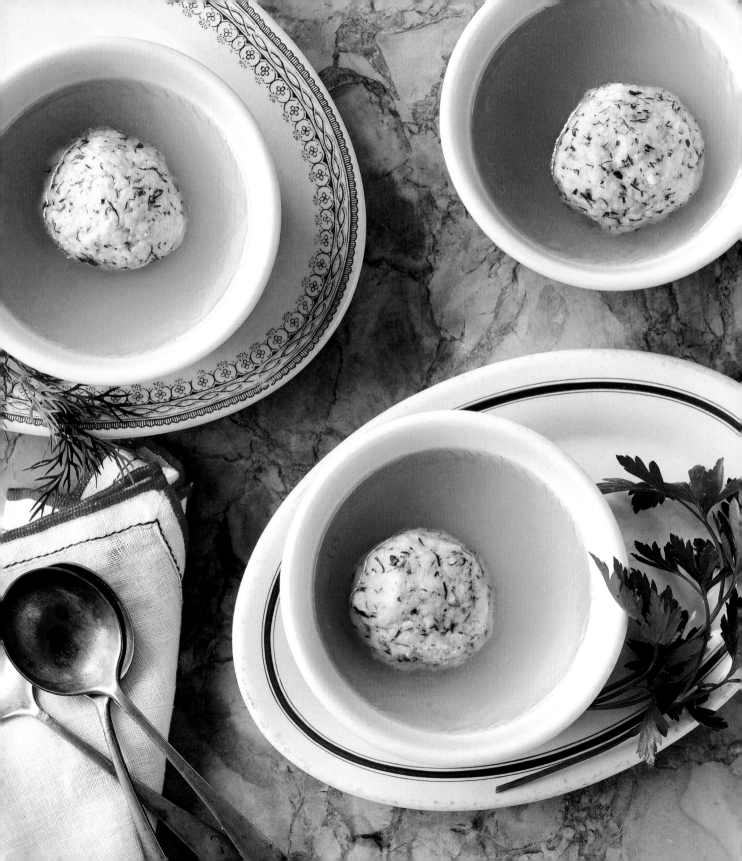

MATZO BALL SOUP

There are two constants at every holiday dinner in my house: It is always very loud—my family doesn't understand the concept of "inside voices"—and there is always matzo ball soup. In fact, it doesn't matter what holiday it is. Be it Passover, Rosh Hashanah, or Thanksgiving, my mother makes matzo ball soup.

Matzo balls are made with matzo meal, a coarsely ground unleavened bread that is traditionally eaten during Passover to commemorate the Israelites' exodus from Egypt. Nowadays, you can find a variety of packaged matzo meals, some of which are kosher for Passover and others which are not. There are even gluten-free versions. The tastiest one, in my opinion, is the Manischewitz brand, which includes some dried seasonings as well as baking soda (sodium bicarbonate) and monocalcium phosphate, both of which work as leavening agents that make the matzo balls soft and fluffy.

My mother's recipe is very simple. All she does is follow the package instructions and add some chopped fresh parsley and dill to the mix. She serves the matzo balls with her chicken soup (see page 71) and garnishes it with more fresh dill and parsley. It's nothing short of delicious and truly makes any day feel like a special occasion.

In a medium bowl, stir together the matzo meal, eggs, avocado oil, water, dill, and parsley with a fork until just combined. Cover the bowl and refrigerate for 20 minutes.

Pour the chicken soup into a medium pot and warm it through over medium-high heat.

Fill a large sauté pan with water (I prefer using a wider pot so the matzo balls have room to expand without getting crowded). Bring the water to a boil and season with 2 tablespoons salt.

¼ cup Manischewitz matzo meal

2 large eggs

2 tablespoons avocado oil

2 tablespoons water or chicken stock

¼ cup loosely packed fresh dill, finely chopped, plus more for garnish

¼ cup loosely packed fresh parsley leaves, finely chopped, plus more for garnish

2 quarts Mama's Chicken Soup (page 71)

Kosher salt

Dairy-Free

Sugar-Free

Time: 35 minutes, plus 20 minutes of chilling

recipe continues

CHICKEN

Wet your hands with some water and roll the matzo meal mixture into golf ball–size balls. Carefully drop the matzo balls into the boiling water, reduce the heat to medium, cover, and cook until you can easily pierce through to the center of a matzo ball with a knife, 20 to 30 minutes. If the matzo balls are still firm, cook for 10 minutes more, then test again; repeat as needed until the matzo balls are tender.

Use a slotted spoon to transfer the matzo balls into individual serving bowls and ladle chicken soup over them. Serve garnished with dill and parsley.

SPICY GREEN BEAN AND CASHEW NUT CHICKEN

This stir-fry comes together in under 15 minutes and uses only a handful of ingredients, making it a perfect back-pocket weeknight dinner. It's great served over a bed of Cauliflower Rice (page 205), but I've eaten it straight out of the pan on more than a few occasions.

Green beans are Whole30-compliant but are technically a legume, which means they're not Paleo. You can, of course, substitute another veggie to suit your individual needs. Asparagus would be a great option because of how similar it is to green beans in shape and color. Other alternatives include thinly sliced zucchini or carrot.

You should also feel free to adjust the amount of red pepper flakes according to your personal preferences. My wife, Catalina, and I both prefer this dish on the spicier side. For an even more interesting kick, try substituting ground Sichuan peppercorns for the red pepper flakes. They fill your mouth with a tingly, numbing sensation that will have you going back for more and more!

In a medium bowl, combine the chicken, coconut aminos, and salt. Toss to coat and set aside to marinate while you prepare the rest of the dish.

Heat a stainless-steel wok or large sauté pan over medium-high heat. Add the avocado oil and heat until it shimmers, about 30 seconds. Add the green beans and cook, stirring, until browned, 3 to 4 minutes. Add the cashews and cook, stirring, until browned, 1 to 2 minutes. Add the garlic and cook, stirring, for 1 minute. Transfer the vegetable-cashew mixture to a bowl and set aside.

3 boneless, skinless chicken breasts (about 12 ounces total), sliced into ⅛-inch-thick strips

¼ cup coconut aminos

¼ teaspoon kosher salt, plus more as needed

2 tablespoons avocado oil

About 7 ounces fresh green beans (substitute asparagus for Paleo), cut into 2-inch pieces (1 cup)

½ cup raw unsalted cashews

2 garlic cloves, finely chopped

1 teaspoon red pepper flakes

2 tablespoons toasted sesame oil

2 cups cooked Cauliflower Rice (page 205)

Gluten-Free
Dairy-Free
Whole30
Grain-Free
Sugar-Free

Time: 20 minutes

recipe continues

CHICKEN

Add the chicken to the pan, reserving the marinade in the bowl. Cook over medium-high heat, stirring, until golden brown and nearly cooked through, 4 to 5 minutes. Return the green beans and cashews to the pan and add the red pepper flakes and reserved marinade. Cook, stirring, until the sauce has reduced by half, 4 to 5 minutes.

Remove the pan from the heat, drizzle in the sesame oil, and toss to coat. Taste and adjust the salt as desired. Serve immediately over the cauliflower rice.

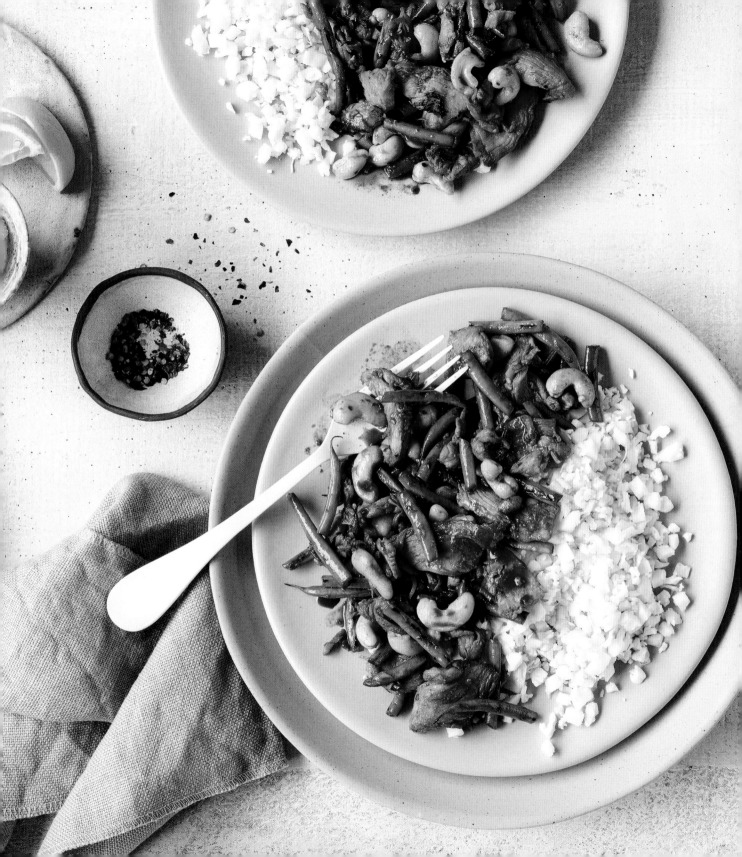

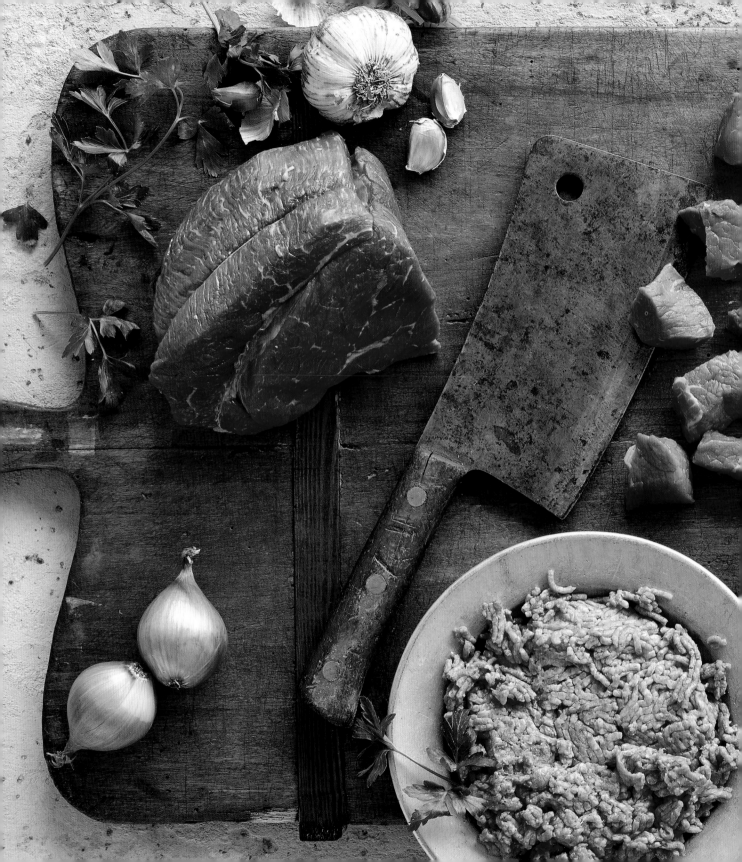

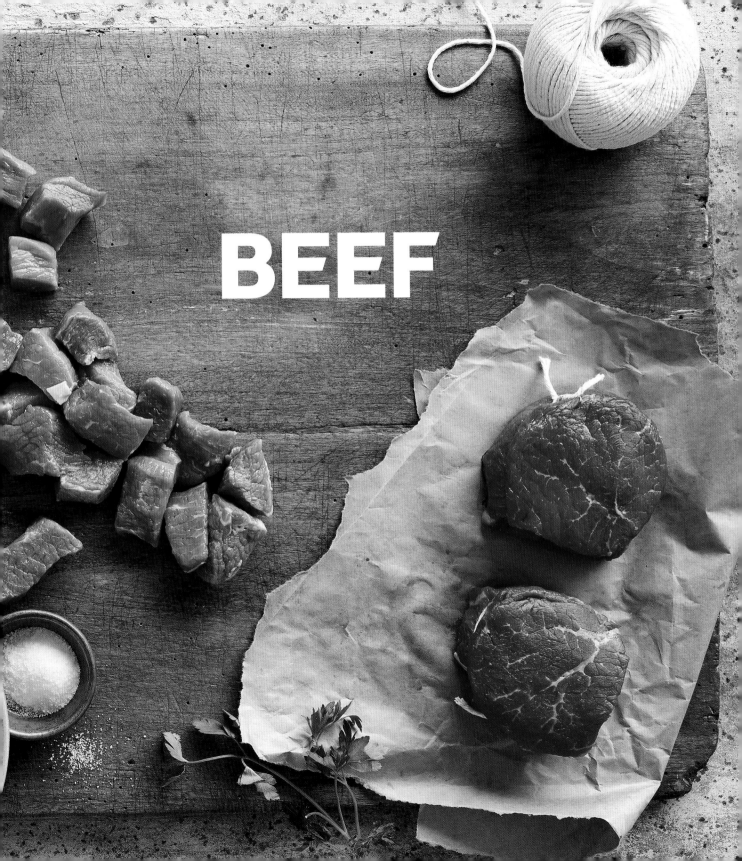

BEEF

CODRUTA'S CIORBA DE VACUTA (ROMANIAN BEEF SOUP)

Gluten-Free

Dairy-Free

Whole30

Grain-Free

Sugar-Free

Time: 2¼ hours

1 pound beef stew meat (preferably chuck; you could also use oxtail or short rib), cut into 2-inch cubes

3 yellow potatoes, peeled and diced

2 carrots, diced

2 parsnips, peeled and diced

1 white onion, diced

1 red bell pepper, diced

Kosher salt

1 tomato

1 tablespoon tomato paste

¼ cup loosely packed fresh lovage or parsley leaves, coarsely chopped, plus more for garnish

Juice of 1 lemon, plus more to taste

1 red onion, thinly sliced, for garnish

I lovingly refer to my mother-in-law as the undisputed queen of soups. Her knowledge and ability to prepare traditional Romanian fare is the stuff of legends. Here I'm sharing her recipe for beef soup, or *ciorba de vacuta* (pronounced *ch-or-buh de vuh-koo-tsa*), which is one of my favorite things to eat. It's hearty, humble, easy to prepare, and incredibly delicious. What sets this beef soup apart from others is the fact that the vegetables are boiled, instead of sautéed, and *bors* is added at the end. Not to be confused with Ukranian or Russian borscht (see page 105), *bors* is a fermented liquid usually made from wheat bran that is often added to different soups to give them a sour note. Because *bors* is hard to find in Toronto, my mother-in-law uses lemon juice instead.

Put the beef in a large pot and add enough water to just cover the meat. Bring to a simmer over medium-high heat, cover, and cook, skimming off any foam that rises to the surface, until the meat is tender, about 1½ hours.

Add the potatoes, carrots, parsnips, onion, and bell pepper. Add more water, if needed, so the liquid reaches just below the top of the pot. Season with salt and bring to a simmer.

Using a sharp knife, score an "X" in the bottom of the tomato. Add the tomato to the soup and cook for 1 minute to loosen the skin. Remove the tomato and run it under cold water. Peel the tomato and discard the skin. Dice the tomato and add it to the soup. Cook until the potatoes are fork-tender, about 20 minutes.

recipe continues

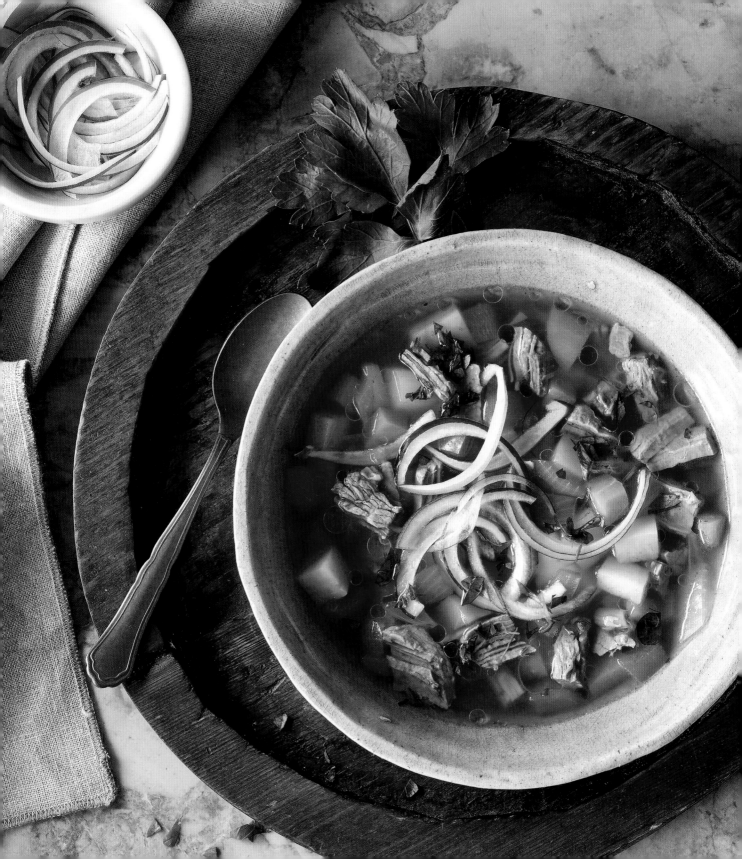

Note: Oxtail is delicious in this soup and adds so much flavor. However, it can take up to 3 hours for the meat to become tender, so if you choose to use oxtail, plan accordingly.

Transfer a ladleful (about ½ cup) of the broth to a small bowl. Stir or whisk in the tomato paste until it has completely dissolved. Add the mixture to the pot and cook for 5 minutes to let the flavors meld.

Stir in the lovage and lemon juice. Taste and adjust the seasoning with additional salt and/or lemon juice as desired—the soup should be slightly sour.

Serve in individual bowls, garnished with the sliced red onion.

STEAK AU POIVRE

Steak au poivre is a classic French bistro dish that typically consists of grilled filet mignon covered in a rich and creamy green peppercorn sauce made with plenty of heavy cream and butter. Here I lighten things up a bit and keep it Whole30-compliant and Paleo-friendly by using ghee and coconut milk. The secret to making things taste as close to the original as possible is to cook down the coconut milk with the shallots. This will mellow the coconut flavor, which might otherwise overpower the dish.

When it comes to cooking the steaks, I'm a big fan of the constant-flip technique, which was popularized by Heston Blumenthal years ago. I have to admit that I resisted it for a very, very long time, preferring instead the tried-and-true flip-once technique. That is, until one fateful day when I was faced with the task of cooking a fairly thick steak without the benefit of an oven and my preferred reverse-sear technique. The result was a perfectly cooked center and evenly caramelized crust. Since then, I've been a convert, but there's a time and place for everything.

There are a few things to consider here. First and foremost, the constant flip works best on bigger steaks, those that are at least 1½ inches thick, because you need time to raise the internal temperature of the meat while simultaneously developing a crust. If your steak is too thin, you will overcook the center before the outside has had a chance to caramelize.

The constant flip also works better for steaks cooked in a well-seasoned cast-iron pan on the stovetop rather than on the grill. Most grill grates are made from stainless steel, to which meat will stick until it develops a crust. Therefore, you are better off only flipping steaks once if you're cooking them on a grill. Well-seasoned cast-iron pans, on the other hand, are virtually nonstick and are more forgiving when it comes to flipping meat before it has developed a crust.

2 (10- to 12-ounce) filets mignons (or substitute your favorite cut such as bavette, rib eye, skirt, porterhouse, flat iron, or New York strip), at least 1½ inches thick

Kosher salt

3 tablespoons avocado oil

1 shallot, finely chopped

¼ cup full-fat coconut milk

½ cup chicken stock

1 tablespoon green peppercorns in brine, drained

1 teaspoon loosely packed fresh thyme leaves, finely chopped

Freshly ground black pepper

1 tablespoon ghee

Gluten-Free

Dairy-Free

Whole30

Keto-Friendly

Paleo

Grain-Free

Sugar-Free

Time: 20 minutes, plus 1 hour of marinating

recipe continues

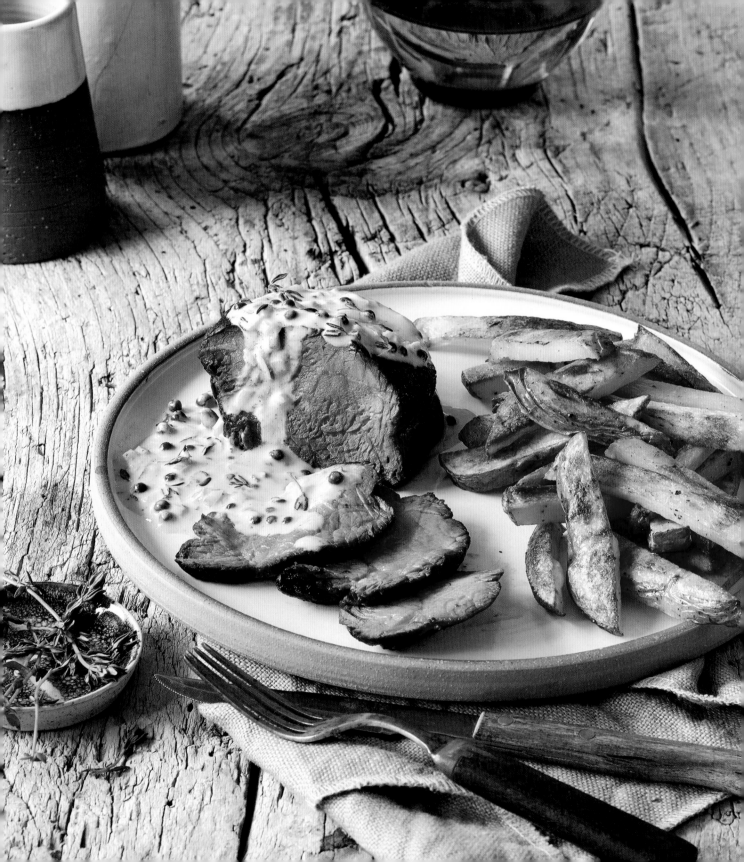

As long as you keep the above considerations in mind, you should have great results using the constant-flip technique when cooking your steak. It safeguards against the fact that all stovetops and skillets perform differently, which can result in one side of the steak cooking more or less than the other.

For a classic French bistro pairing, serve this steak with my Oven Fries (page 200).

Pat the steaks dry with paper towels and liberally season all sides with salt. Place on a rimmed baking sheet and set aside for 1 hour at room temperature.

When ready to cook the steaks, heat a large cast-iron skillet over medium heat for 5 minutes. Increase the heat to medium-high and pour in 2 tablespoons of the avocado oil. Heat until oil is shimmering and carefully place the steaks in the skillet. Cook, flipping the steaks every 60 seconds, until the internal temperature registers 130° to 135°F on an instant-read thermometer, about 8 minutes. Remove the steaks from the pan and transfer them to a wire rack to rest for 10 minutes.

While the steaks rest, wipe the skillet clean with a paper towel, then place it over medium heat. Pour in the remaining 1 tablespoon avocado oil, then add the shallot. Cook, stirring, until softened, 1 to 2 minutes. Stir in the coconut milk and cook, stirring occasionally, until the liquid has reduced by about half, about 2 minutes.

Add the stock, green peppercorns, thyme, and a pinch of black pepper. Cook until the sauce has reduced again by half, about 4 minutes. Fold in the ghee and stir until it has melted. Taste the sauce and season with salt and pepper as desired.

Slice the steaks against the grain and arrange them on a serving platter. Spoon the green peppercorn sauce over the top and serve.

STIR-FRIED BEEF
WITH MUSHROOMS, ZUCCHINI, AND BEAN SPROUTS

Gluten-Free

Dairy-Free

Whole30

Paleo

Grain-Free

Sugar-Free

Time: 15 minutes

2 top sirloin medallions (about 8 ounces total), sliced very thinly against the grain

2 tablespoons avocado oil

1 cup (8 ounces) thinly sliced cremini or white button mushrooms

½ yellow onion, sliced

Kosher salt

1 zucchini, sliced into half-moons

1 jalapeño, seeded and thinly sliced (optional)

2 garlic cloves, thinly sliced

1 cup (8 ounces) bean sprouts

¼ cup coconut aminos

½ teaspoon fish sauce

2 scallions, white and light green parts only, sliced into 2-inch pieces

1 tablespoon toasted sesame oil

1 tablespoon sesame seeds, for garnish

Here's a quick-and-easy 15-minute meal (cooking time) that is perfect for those days when you don't want to do any heavy lifting in the kitchen. It's also a great way to utilize cheaper cuts of meat like top sirloin, flat iron, or even top sirloin medallions, which are a hidden gem because unlike top sirloin, the medallions are free of any gristle and perfect for stir-fries! Try serving the beef over some Cauliflower Rice (page 205), or steamed rice, if you're living your Food Freedom.

You can make this stir-fry in your favorite wok, stainless-steel sauté pan, or even a cast-iron skillet. Most people own at least one stainless-steel pan, so that's what I used here.

Tips for stir-frying in stainless steel:

1. Gradually preheat the pan over medium-low heat before adding the oil.
2. Preheat the oil before adding the meat.
3. Cook the meat without stirring until it forms a crust. Only then should you try to flip or stir the meat.
4. Keep the heat on at least medium-high throughout the cooking process. Otherwise, you run the risk of steaming instead of stir-frying. I like to cook this on the highest heat possible, but this will depend on the strength of your stovetop. Gas, coil, and induction ranges are far more powerful than electric burners.
5. Prep all the ingredients ahead of time. This dish comes together quickly, especially over high heat, so it's important to be ready to roll.

Pat the beef very dry with paper towels and set aside on a plate.

Heat a large stainless-steel sauté pan over medium heat for
5 minutes. Increase the heat to high, pour in the avocado oil, and
heat until shimmering. Working in batches, add the beef and
cook until browned, about 4 minutes, being careful not to over-
crowd the pan. Transfer the cooked beef to a bowl and repeat to
brown the remaining beef. You may notice that the beef bubbles
and releases excess moisture as it browns; simply cook until it
evaporates.

Reduce the heat to medium and add the mushrooms and onion.
Season with salt and cook, stirring regularly to avoid burning, until
softened, 3 to 4 minutes. Add the zucchini and jalapeño (if using)
and cook, stirring, for 2 minutes. Add the garlic and cook, stirring, for
1 minute. Add the bean sprouts, coconut aminos, and fish sauce and
cook, stirring occasionally, until the sauce has reduced by half, about
5 minutes.

Remove the pan from the heat. Return the beef to the pan and add
the scallions and sesame oil. Toss everything to coat. Garnish with
the sesame seeds and serve immediately.

ROAST SHORT RIBS
WITH ZHUG, TAHINI, AND ALMONDS

Gluten-Free

Dairy-Free

Whole30

Keto-Friendly

Paleo

Grain-Free

Sugar-Free

Time: 3 hours, plus 4 hours of marinating

6 English-cut bone-in beef short ribs (about 3 pounds total)

Kosher salt and freshly ground black pepper

¼ cup slivered toasted almonds, for serving

½ cup Zhug (page 246), for serving

½ cup Tahini Sauce (page 240), for serving

2 lemons, cut into wedges, for serving

One of my favorite techniques for achieving incredibly moist, succulent, fork-tender beef ribs is to roast them low and slow in the oven with a splash of water. As the water heats, it creates a steamy environment for the beef to cook in. Slowly, the water evaporates and allows the meat to caramelize from the dry heat of the oven. The result is a perfectly juicy and tender rib with a crispy crust. It's nothing short of magic.

Make sure you choose a well-marbled cut of meat, such as short rib or chuck roast, which won't dry out, unlike top sirloin or eye of round, and doesn't require any additional cooking fat. As far as flavors go, I've kept things very simple. The meat is very rich and can hold its own with just a bit of salt and pepper, especially since the tahini, zhug, and almonds bring a lot of flavor to the table. For more oomph, try rubbing the ribs with a combination of dry spices commonly used in Middle Eastern cooking. Think toasted cumin seed, coriander seed, fenugreek, paprika, cayenne pepper, cinnamon, etc. The possibilities are truly endless!

Not a fan of beef? Try this same method for making my Jerk Ribs (page 142), roasted lamb shanks with rosemary and garlic, or pork shoulder with achiote paste for a wonderful Cochinita Pibil (page 143).

Like the Roast Cauliflower on page 203, this recipe is inspired by an amazing dish that Catalina and I enjoyed at Miznon, in the Vienna location. One of the specials the day we ate there was a giant slow-roasted beef rib. I remember the taste like it was yesterday: rich, succulent, fork-tender, melt-in-your-mouth beefy goodness. We smothered it in a house-made fiery green Yemeni hot sauce called *zhug*. The combination of flavors, colors, and textures is not one I'll soon forget!

Pat the short ribs dry with paper towels and place them on a rimmed baking sheet. Liberally season them on all sides with salt and pepper. Cover and refrigerate for at least 4 hours or up to overnight.

When ready to cook the ribs, preheat the oven to 350°F.

Pat the short ribs dry with paper towels and place them in a roasting pan. Pour in ½ cup water. Cover the pan tightly with aluminum foil and roast the ribs for 2½ to 3 hours, until the meat is extremely tender and can be easily shredded with a fork. Larger cuts will take slightly longer to cook; if the meat is not tender after 3 hours, cover the pan again and cook for 30 minutes more, then check again; repeat until the meat is tender.

Meanwhile, in a small skillet, toast the almonds over medium-low heat until warmed through and fragrant, about 5 minutes.

Transfer the short ribs to a serving platter and drizzle with the zhug and tahini sauce. Squeeze the lemon wedges over the top, garnish with the toasted almonds, and serve.

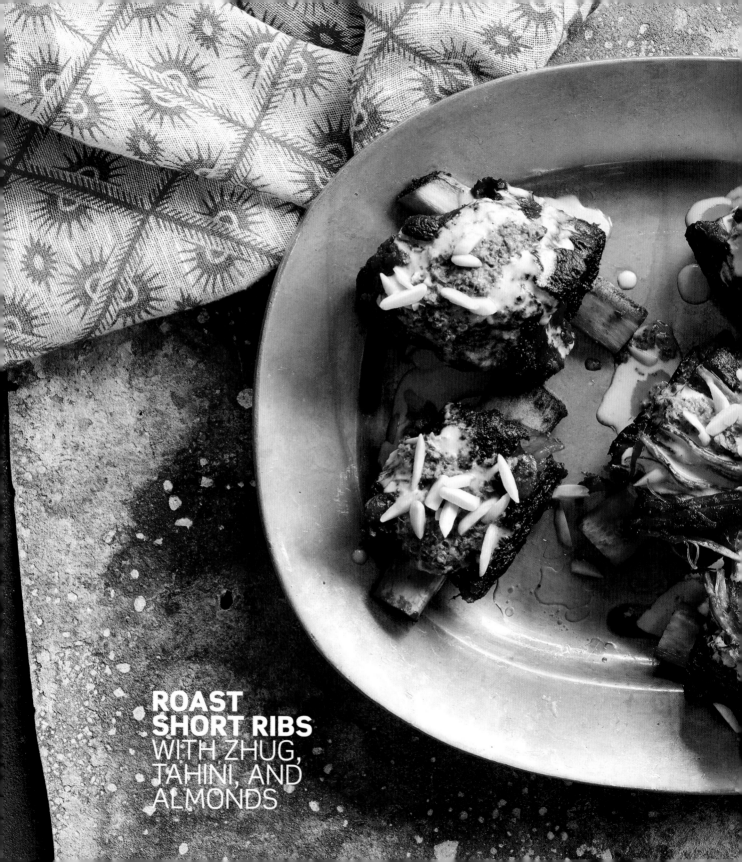

**ROAST
SHORT RIBS**
WITH ZHUG,
TAHINI, AND
ALMONDS

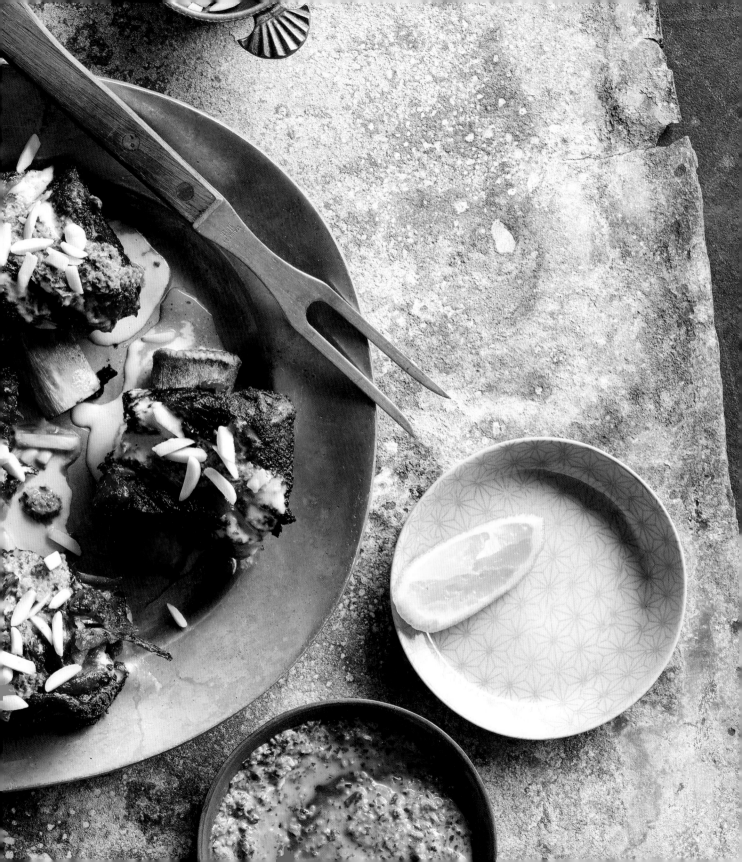

PICADILLO

Gluten-Free

Dairy-Free

Whole30

Keto-Friendly

Paleo

Grain-Free

Sugar-Free

Time: 1 hour

1 tablespoon avocado oil

2 pounds lean ground beef

1 large yellow onion, thinly sliced

1 red bell pepper, diced

5 garlic cloves, finely chopped

2 teaspoons smoked Spanish paprika

2 teaspoons ancho chile powder

1 teaspoon ground cumin

1 teaspoon dried oregano

1 teaspoon kosher salt, plus more as needed

1 teaspoon freshly ground black pepper, plus more as needed

1½ cups chicken stock

1½ cups sliced pitted green olives, such as Manzanilla

¼ cup no-sugar-added dark raisins (optional)

2 bay leaves

Picadillo, from the Spanish word *picar*, meaning "mince," is a common dish found throughout South America and the Philippines made with ground meat, usually beef. This version is a riff on the Cuban staple that I regularly enjoyed when visiting my grandparents in Miami. The smoked paprika and ancho chile powder may not be "traditional," but they add a wonderful depth of flavor. Personally, I prefer my picadillo without raisins, but you're the boss, applesauce. Try serving it over some Cauliflower Rice (page 205), or steamed rice if you're living your Food Freedom, and with a side of Twice-Fried Plantains (page 218) or Sweet Plantains (Maduros) (page 210).

In a large Dutch oven or heavy-bottomed pot, heat the avocado oil over medium-high heat. Working in batches, add the ground beef and cook, breaking it up with your spoon as it cooks, until browned, about 12 minutes. Transfer the beef to a bowl and repeat to cook the remaining meat.

Discard all but 2 tablespoons of the rendered fat from the pot and set it over medium heat. Add the onion and bell pepper and cook, stirring, until the onion is slightly caramelized, 8 to 10 minutes. Add the garlic and cook, stirring, until fragrant, about 1 minute. Add the paprika, ancho chile powder, cumin, oregano, salt, and black pepper. Stir, letting the spices warm and toast, for 1 minute. Add the stock and stir, using your spoon to scrape up any browned bits from the bottom of the pot.

Return the beef to the pot and add the olives, raisins (if using), and bay leaves. Increase the heat to medium-high and bring the sauce to a simmer. Reduce the heat to low, cover, and cook, stirring occasionally to prevent burning, until the beef is tender, at least 30 minutes or up to 1 hour for a more intensely flavored finished product. Taste and season with additional salt and pepper as desired. Discard the bay leaves. Let stand 10 minutes before serving.

Notes: If your picadillo is a bit too watery, remove the lid and cook for 5 to 10 minutes more to allow some of the moisture in the pot to evaporate. This will also concentrate the rich flavors of the picadillo—a good thing! You are aiming for a thick yet juicy consistency that loosely coats the back of a spoon. Just be careful not to reduce the sauce for much longer than 10 minutes, or it may dry out or burn.

You can make picadillo the day before and reheat it at the time of serving. The flavors will continue to develop in the refrigerator overnight and it will taste even better the next day! If it seems too dry the following day, simply add a bit of chicken stock or water.

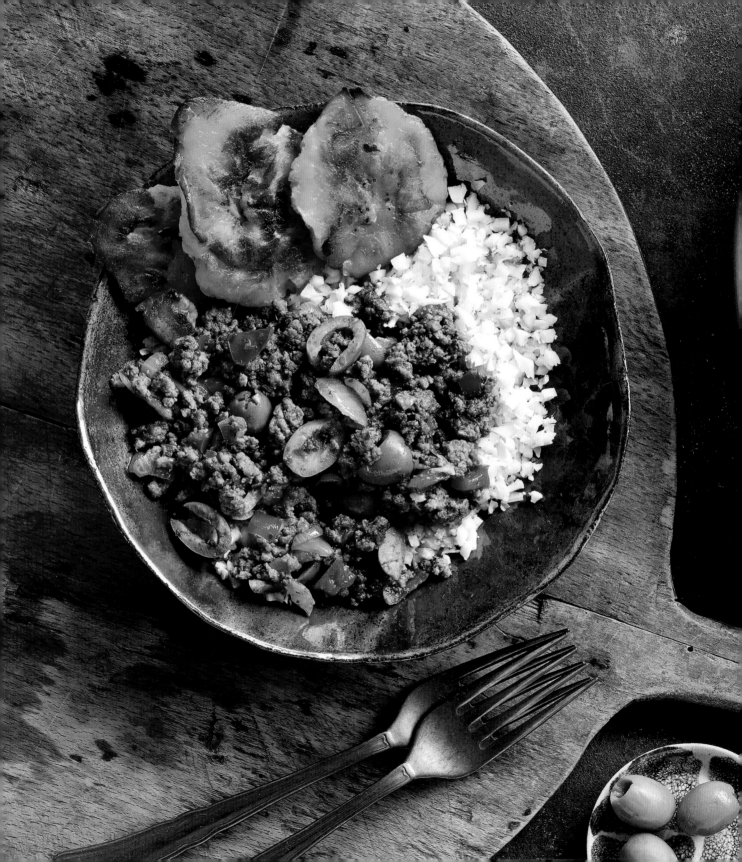

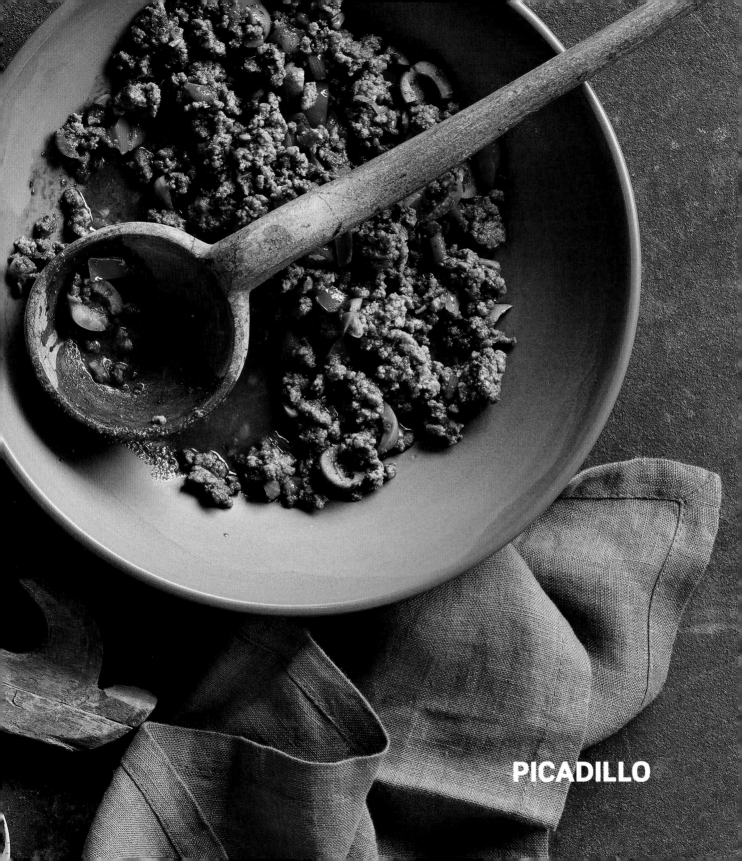

PICADILLO

MICI

Gluten-Free
Dairy-Free
Whole30
Keto-Friendly
Paleo
Grain-Free
Sugar-Free

Time: 20 minutes,
plus at least
6 hours of
marinating

2 pounds lean ground beef

1 pound ground pork

½ cup carbonated mineral water

4 garlic cloves, minced

1 tablespoon kosher salt, plus more for seasoning

2 teaspoons baking soda

1 teaspoon dried oregano

1 teaspoon freshly ground black pepper

¼ cup Dijon mustard, for serving

Mici (pronounced *mee-tch*), meaning "small" in Romanian, are log-shaped ground meat kebabs typically grilled over charcoal. It used to be that you could find *mici* vendors at just about every major street corner, beside bus stops, and outside train stations and grocery stores. These days, it has become more and more difficult to find the Romanian version of the hot dog or kebab cart. You may still come across the occasional vendor at a local market, but it seems that this street food has slowly made its way indoors and onto the menus of restaurants that now charge a premium for it.

My father-in-law, a veritable *mici* connoisseur, tells me that many traditional recipes call for using beef exclusively. However, as prepackaged ground meat has become more and more geared toward those looking for leaner options, it became popular to lace the beef with a fattier grind of pork, lamb, or mutton to make sure the finished product isn't dry. If you can find medium-fatty ground beef, such as chuck, which is 80 to 85% fat, you can probably get away with using it exclusively, which is a great option for those who keep kosher or halal. Otherwise, feel free to combine two parts ground beef with one part fattier ground meat, such as pork.

Regardless of the meat mixture, my father-in-law tells me that there are a few things you cannot do without. The first is garlic, the defining flavor in *mici*. The second is the addition of baking soda, which makes the *mici* light and airy. Last but not least, you will want to add some water, which seems counterintuitive but also makes for a more delicate and juicy *mici*. If you ask my mother-in-law, she'll insist you use carbonated mineral water. My father-in-law, on the other hand, says you can use flat water. For even more flavor and juiciness, try adding a bit of gelatinous beef or pork bone broth in place of the water.

In a large bowl, combine the ground beef, ground pork, carbonated water, garlic, salt, baking soda, oregano, and pepper. Use your hands

recipe continues

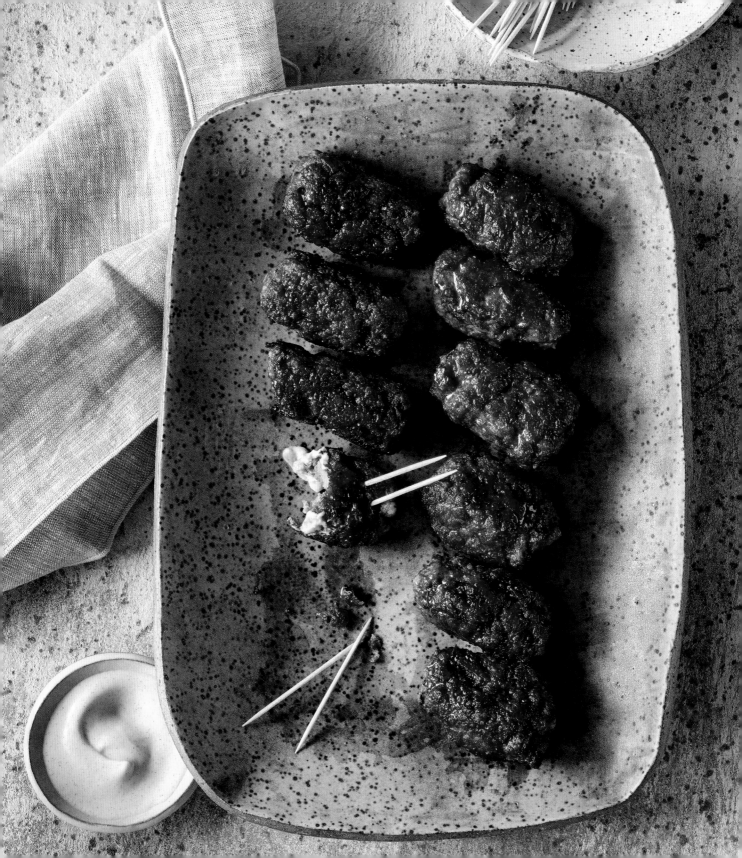

to thoroughly mix until the mixture is tacky and well combined. Test the seasoning by frying a tablespoon of the mixture in a dry nonstick skillet over medium-high heat. Taste the cooked portion and season the raw mixture with salt as needed. Cover the bowl with plastic wrap and refrigerate for at least 6 hours or up to overnight.

Line a baking sheet with parchment paper. Using your hands, form small, log-shaped kebabs approximately 3½ inches long and 1 inch thick, placing them on the baking sheet as you form them.

Heat a grill to medium-high (a charcoal grill is ideal, though gas is fine, too) or heat a cast-iron grill pan over medium-high heat. Grill the mici until browned and cooked through, 3 to 4 minutes per side.

Serve immediately, with toothpicks for picking up the mici and mustard for dipping.

SHORT RIB RAGÙ

Using bone-in short ribs will deliver the most flavor in this ragù, but boneless will cook a bit quicker. An electronic or stovetop pressure cooker will also save you some time and can be a lifesaver if you're in a hurry. However, I encourage you to first try making this short rib ragù the old-fashioned way, on the stovetop. It's hard to beat a ragù that has had a chance to slowly reduce and concentrate in flavor as moisture evaporates and escapes the pot.

Try tossing the ragù with some Perfect Zucchini Noodles (page 188) or serving it over a bed of fluffy cauliflower grits (see page 162). If you're living your Food Freedom, I recommend going with a rigatoni or pappardelle, gluten-free or regular, or serving the ragù over some corn polenta, which is also gluten-free.

Heat a Dutch oven or electric pressure cooker over medium-high heat for 5 minutes. Pat the short ribs very dry with paper towels and generously season them on all sides with salt. Increase the heat to medium-high and pour in the avocado oil. Heat the oil until shimmering, add the short ribs in batches, and cook until browned, 3 to 4 minutes on each side. Transfer the browned meat to a bowl and set aside.

Reduce the heat to medium and add the celery, carrots, and onion to the pot. Season with a pinch of salt. Cook, stirring and scraping up all the browned bits from the bottom of the pot, until the vegetables are softened, 10 to 12 minutes. Stir in the garlic and cook, stirring, for 1 minute.

Return the browned meat to the pot and add the tomato puree, thyme, and bay leaves. Season with ½ teaspoon each of salt and pepper, stir to combine, and bring the sauce to a simmer. Reduce the heat to low, cover, and cook until the meat is fall-apart tender,

2 pounds English-cut bone-in beef short ribs

Kosher salt

1 tablespoon avocado oil

3 celery stalks, diced

2 carrots, diced

1 yellow onion, diced

12 garlic cloves, smashed and peeled

2 (24-ounce) cans or jars tomato puree (see page 239)

6 sprigs thyme

2 bay leaves

Freshly ground black pepper

Handful of fresh basil leaves, torn

Gluten-Free

Dairy-Free

Whole30

Keto-Friendly

Paleo

Grain-Free

Sugar-Free

Time: 3½ hours

recipe continues

BEEF

2½ to 3 hours. If using a pressure cooker, lock on the lid and cook on HIGH pressure for 1½ hours. If the ragù has reduced too much or becomes clumpy, simply add a little bit of stock to thin it out. It should coat the back of a spoon.

Transfer the meat to a bowl and shred it with two forks. Discard the bones, thyme sprigs, and bay leaves. If you're using a pressure cooker, you may want to reduce the sauce briefly over medium-low heat with the pot uncovered, depending on your tastes and the consistency of the sauce.

Return the shredded meat to the pot and stir in the basil. Taste and adjust the seasoning as desired. Serve immediately.

BRONIA'S BORSCHT

While most of my friends would ask their grandparents for toys, bikes, or money to play at the arcade, all I ever wanted was my babushka Bronia's borscht and to spend time with my *dedushka* Michael.

Some of my fondest memories are ones visiting my grandparents in Miami. There would be five of us all crowded into a one-bedroom apartment. My brother and I would sleep on air mattresses, and my mother would take the fold-out sofa bed. My grandfather, a retired master jeweler, was still so in love with his craft that he had set up a "workshop" in the tiny closet in their bedroom. For hours on end, I would sit and watch him effortlessly apply filigree, engrave gold, and set diamonds and gemstones by hand. His tireless work ethic was matched only by his endless patience, positivity, and kindness. He was one of those rare souls whom absolutely everyone loved to be around.

If I wasn't in my grandfather's "workshop," I was in the kitchen with my grandmother. It was a tight and claustrophobic space with 7-foot drop-ceilings and no ventilation. With virtually no space on the countertop, my grandmother would sit at the half-moon kitchen table and prepare all the meals with the world's smallest paring knife and cutting board. I have vivid memories of being in that kitchen and watching her cook things like buckwheat with fried onions, sautéed chicken liver, and her specialty, borscht. All the while, beads of sweat slowly dripped down my brow from the intense steam and wonky air conditioner.

My grandmother's borscht is a Ukrainian one, deep red in color with plenty of beets, cabbage, potatoes, and beef and served piping hot. Aside from the immense amount of love she put into every pot, there are a few things that made her version insanely delicious. She always used bone-in beef short rib for its fat and flavor and added some white sugar to balance the acidity from the vinegar, which she added at the end. The soup was always hearty, rich, and perfectly balanced in flavor and texture.

2 pounds cross-cut beef short ribs, cut into pieces between the bones

3 bay leaves

Kosher salt

1 teaspoon whole black peppercorns

2 tablespoons avocado oil

1½ pounds beets, grated

3 carrots, grated

1 yellow onion, coarsely chopped

1 (6-ounce) can tomato paste

2 pounds white potatoes, peeled and cut into 2-inch cubes

1 large parsnip, peeled and diced

1 small green cabbage, thinly sliced

Juice of 1 lemon, plus more if needed

Freshly ground black pepper

¼ cup loosely packed fresh dill leaves, coarsely chopped

¼ cup loosely packed fresh parsley leaves, coarsely chopped

Gluten-Free
Dairy-Free
Whole30
Grain-Free
Sugar-Free

Time: 3 hours

recipe continues

BEEF

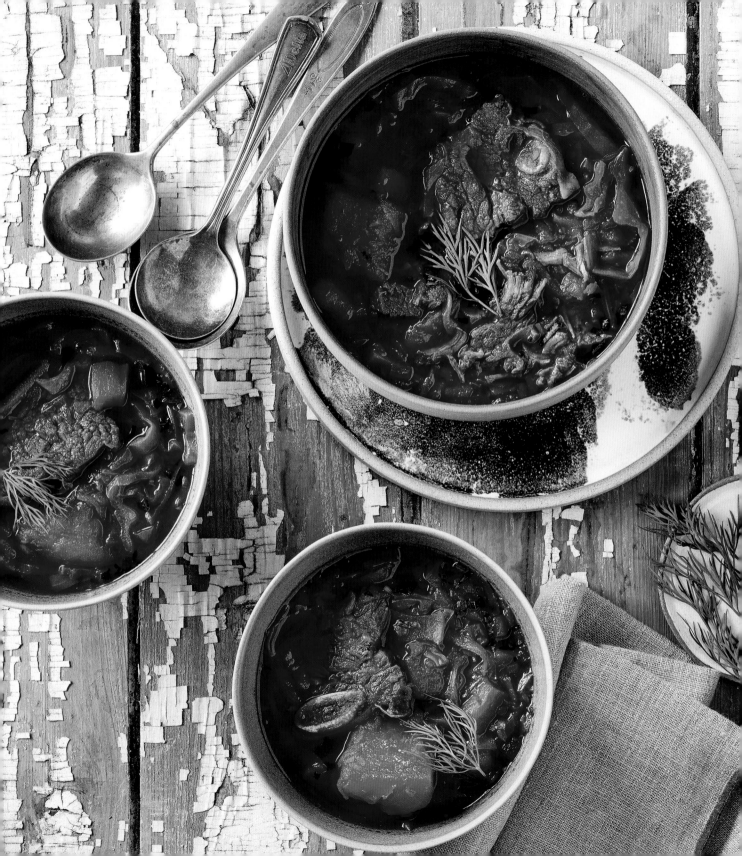

Interestingly enough, only a few minor adjustments are necessary to make her recipe Whole30-compliant. It's as simple as using avocado oil in place of the vegetable oil and omitting the sugar, which is not essential because the carrots, onion, and beets in the soup are sweet enough. I also omit the sour cream that is customarily dolloped onto the borscht before serving, but if you're living your Food Freedom, you can certainly give it a try. It adds a subtle tang and creaminess that is truly delicious. I don't think my grandmother would mind either way.

In a very large stockpot or Dutch oven, combine the ribs, bay leaves, 2 tablespoons salt, and the peppercorns. Add enough water to cover the ribs and bring to a boil over high heat. Reduce the heat to maintain a steady simmer, cover, and cook, skimming off any foam that rises to the surface, until the meat is falling off the bone, 1½ to 2 hours.

While the ribs cook, in a 4-quart stockpot, heat the avocado oil over medium heat. Add the beets, carrots, and onion and season with a pinch of salt. Cook, stirring often, until the vegetables are tender, about 12 minutes. Add the tomato paste and cook, stirring to coat the vegetables, until thickened, about 3 minutes. Remove from the heat and set aside.

When the ribs are tender and the meat is falling off the bone, add the potatoes and parsnip to the pot and cook until fork-tender, about 25 minutes. Reduce the heat to low, stir in the beet-carrot mixture, and cook until the broth has turned red, about 10 minutes. Add the cabbage and lemon juice and cook until the cabbage is slightly softened, about 10 minutes.

Taste the borscht and season with salt, pepper, or lemon juice as desired—it should taste sweet and sour. Remove from the heat and stir in the dill and parsley. Let the soup stand for 10 minutes before serving.

HAMBURGER SOUP

Gluten-Free
Dairy-Free
Whole30
Grain-Free
Sugar-Free

Time: 1 hour, plus
30 minutes of
resting

1 tablespoon extra-
virgin olive oil

1 pound lean
ground beef

3 celery stalks, diced
(about 1½ cups)

3 carrots, diced
(about 1½ cups)

1 red onion, diced

1 red bell pepper,
diced

Kosher salt

4 garlic cloves,
finely chopped

4 cups beef stock

1 (28-ounce) can
crushed tomatoes
(I like San Marzano)

3 yellow potatoes,
peeled, if desired,
and cubed

2 bay leaves

1 tablespoon fresh
thyme leaves

½ teaspoon freshly
ground black pepper,
plus more as needed

2 cups frozen
chopped green beans

½ cup thinly sliced dill
pickles, for garnish

Hamburger soup is an easy, hearty, delicious one-pot meal that will feed a crowd. It's best prepared ahead of time so the flavors have a chance to get to know each other. The soup can also be frozen in individual servings and reheated on the stovetop for those days when you don't have the time or energy to cook from scratch. I actually made a big batch of this soup before my wife went into labor, and it couldn't have been better on those cold, sleepless winter nights after our baby was born.

Feel free to use just about any vegetable you want or have on hand. I've kept things pretty simple here, but you could just as easily add cauliflower, broccoli, zucchini, eggplant, or leeks, to name just a few. Using frozen vegetables is a real time-saver here because it frees you from having to rinse and chop.

No matter what ingredients you choose to include, I strongly encourage you to top your Hamburger Soup with some chopped pickles. Like any good burger, this soup just isn't the same without them!

In a large Dutch oven or heavy-bottomed stockpot, heat the olive oil over medium-high heat. Working in batches, add the ground beef and cook, breaking up the meat with a wooden spoon as it cooks, until browned, 10 to 12 minutes. Using a slotted spoon, transfer the beef to a bowl and repeat to brown the remaining beef.

Discard all but 2 tablespoons of the rendered fat from the pot. Return the pot to medium heat and add the celery, carrots, onion, and bell pepper. Season with salt. Cook the vegetables for 2 to 3 minutes, using a wooden spoon to scrape up any browned bits from the bottom of the pot. Add the garlic and cook, stirring, for 1 minute.

Return the browned beef back to the pot and add the stock, crushed tomatoes, potatoes, bay leaves, thyme, pepper, and 2 cups water. Bring to a boil over high heat, then reduce the heat to medium-low, cover, and cook at a steady simmer, stirring occasionally to prevent burning, for 30 minutes. Add the green beans and cook until they are warmed through, 2 to 3 minutes. Taste and adjust the seasoning.

For best results, let the soup cool in the pot for about 30 minutes before serving. Ladle into individual bowls, top with slices of dill pickle, and serve.

STEAK OSCAR

Gluten-Free

Dairy-Free

Whole30

Keto-Friendly

Paleo

Grain-Free

Sugar-Free

Time: 40 minutes,
plus 1 hour of
resting

For the Steaks and Shrimp:

2 (10- to 12-ounce) filets mignons (or substitute your favorite cut such as bavette, rib eye, skirt, porterhouse, flat iron, or New York strip), roughly 2 inches thick

Kosher salt

10 asparagus spears, woody ends trimmed

3 tablespoons avocado oil

Freshly ground black pepper

6 raw jumbo black tiger shrimp, peeled, tails kept on, and deveined

1 tablespoon Adobo Seasoning (page 254)

For the Hollandaise:

½ cup ghee or grass-fed butter

1 large egg yolk

1 teaspoon fresh lemon juice

Pinch of kosher salt

1 tablespoon fresh tarragon leaves, finely chopped

Think of this as more of a road map than a recipe. There are a lot of twists and turns you can make before reaching your delicious destination. For starters, feel free to use just about any steak you like! The original version of this dish is believed to have been created for King Oscar II of Sweden using veal medallions. These days it's more common to find it served with filet mignon (beef tenderloin). For a lowbrow, albeit delicious, substitution, try top-sirloin medallions. Truth be told, many different cuts will do (New York strip, rib eye, flat iron, bavette, porterhouse, Denver, etc.). Heck, you could even use chicken breast if so desired! Just keep in mind that the hollandaise sauce is very rich, so it may be best to pair it with leaner cuts of meat.

Speaking of sauce, béarnaise was likely what King Oscar II was served. However, hollandaise is just as delicious and a bit easier to prepare, especially when using the technique outlined here (adapted from J. Kenji López-Alt's book *The Food Lab*).

As far as cooking the steak goes, I'm a fan of the constant-flip technique (see Steak au Poivre, page 87). When it comes to toppings, asparagus is a common denominator, but the options are truly endless. Grilled bell peppers, sautéed green beans, or even broccoli florets would go great here. Last but not least, feel free to substitute crabmeat for the shrimp. Or if you're feeling a bit extravagant, use both!

MAKE THE STEAKS AND SHRIMP: Pat the steaks very dry with paper towels and liberally season all sides with salt. Place on a baking sheet and set aside for 1 hour.

Meanwhile, fill a large bowl with ice and water and set it nearby.

Bring a large stainless-steel pot of water to a boil over medium-high heat. Season the water with a pinch of salt, add the asparagus, and cook until bright green and just tender, about 2 minutes. Transfer to the ice water and let cool for 5 minutes, then drain thoroughly. Set aside.

recipe continues

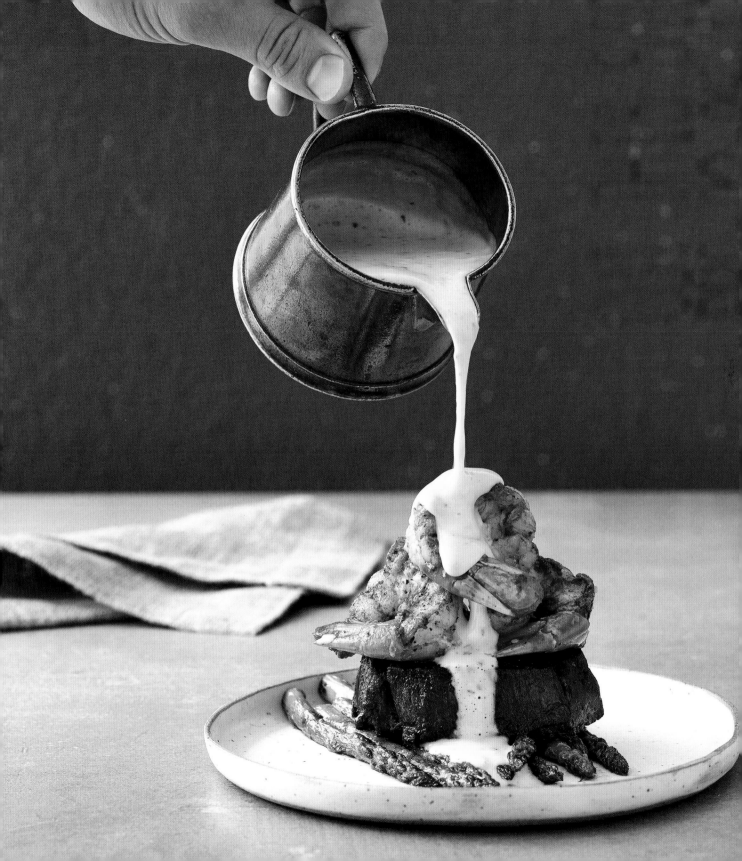

Heat a large cast-iron skillet over medium heat for 5 minutes. Increase the heat to medium-high and add 2 tablespoons of the avocado oil. Heat the oil until it shimmers, and then carefully lay the steaks in the skillet and cook, flipping them every 60 seconds, until the internal temperature registers 130° to 135°F (medium-rare to medium) on an instant-read thermometer, about 8 minutes. Transfer the steaks to a wire rack, lightly season with pepper, and let rest for 10 minutes.

Wipe the skillet clean, return it to medium-high heat, and add the remaining 1 tablespoon avocado oil. In a medium bowl, combine the shrimp and the adobo seasoning and toss to coat. Add the shrimp to the hot oil and cook until golden brown and cooked through, 2 to 3 minutes per side. Transfer the shrimp to a plate and set aside.

Add the blanched asparagus to the pan and toss until warmed through, about 2 minutes.

MAKE THE HOLLANDAISE: In a small saucepan, melt the ghee over medium heat. Transfer the melted ghee to a measuring cup or small bowl with a spout.

In a widemouthed mason jar, combine the egg yolk, lemon juice, salt, and 1 teaspoon water. Center the head of the immersion blender over the egg yolk and blend on the lowest speed (if your blender has multiple speeds), without moving the blender, for about 10 seconds. With the blender running, slowly stream in the melted ghee until the sauce is emulsified, about 1 minute. If you accidentally overwork the hollandaise sauce and it becomes too thick, simply add a teaspoon or two of warm water and blend until it becomes smooth and creamy again. Add the tarragon and stir through to combine.

To serve, divide the asparagus between two plates, arranging the spears in an even layer. Top each with a steak, divide the shrimp between them, and pour or spoon the hollandaise over the top.

ZHARKOE

Zharkoe (pronounced *zhar-koh-yuh*) is a very simple stew most often made with beef and potatoes. You will find a pot of this slowly bubbling away in a *kazan* (cauldron) on the stove of just about every Russian or Ukrainian household. And everyone who makes it has a slightly different recipe. Some use a tomato product to make the broth; others, like my parents, don't.

Though any type of stew meat will work here, I recommend using something with a decent amount of fat, such as chuck. The marbling in the meat will not only add a tremendous amount of flavor to the stew, but will also prevent it from drying out, which will happen if you use a leaner cut, such as eye of round.

Zharkoe is, in my opinion, one of the finest examples of peasant food, a humble dish that is born out of necessity yet so incredibly filling and unbelievably delicious. It requires some patience and a bit of work in the kitchen, but as with most things in life, the reward is well worth the effort.

In a Dutch oven or heavy-bottomed pot, heat the avocado oil over medium-high heat. Add the beef and cook, stirring regularly, until browned on all sides and all the moisture has evaporated, about 15 minutes. Add the onions, carrots, salt, and pepper and cook, stirring and scraping up any browned bits from the bottom of the pan, until the vegetables have started to caramelize, 8 to 10 minutes. Add the garlic and cook, stirring, for 1 minute.

Add enough water to barely cover the meat and bring the liquid to a simmer. Reduce the heat to medium-low, cover, and cook, stirring occasionally, until the beef is soft, 1½ to 2 hours. If at any point the liquid evaporates enough that the meat is exposed, add water as needed to just barely cover the beef.

Add the potatoes and enough water to cover the contents of the pot. Cook until the potatoes are soft, 25 to 30 minutes. Taste and adjust the seasoning. Let cool for 5 minutes before serving.

2 tablespoons avocado oil

2 pounds beef stew meat, such as chuck, cut into 2-inch pieces

3 yellow onions (about 1 pound), diced

4 small carrots (about 10 ounces total), cut into rounds

2 teaspoons kosher salt, plus more as needed

1 tablespoon freshly ground black pepper, plus more as needed

3 garlic cloves, coarsely chopped

1 pound yellow potatoes (about 4), peeled and cut into 3-inch-long wedges

Gluten-Free

Dairy-Free

Whole30

Grain-Free

Sugar-Free

Time: 3 hours

CATALINA'S GROUND MEAT TACOS

THE PRIMAL GOURMET COOKBOOK

Gluten-Free

Dairy-Free

Whole30

Keto-Friendly

Paleo

Grain-Free

Sugar-Free

Time: 1½ hours

1⅔ cups chicken stock

1 dried ancho chile

1 dried New Mexico chile

1 tablespoon avocado oil

2 pounds ground beef (80 to 85% lean ground beef is preferred but leaner ground beef will work as well)

1 yellow onion, diced

¾ teaspoon kosher salt, plus more as needed

5 garlic cloves, finely chopped

1 tablespoon granulated onion

1 teaspoon hot paprika

1 teaspoon ground cumin

1 teaspoon dried oregano, preferably Mexican

There are two things I cook for my wife, Catalina, when I'm in the doghouse. The first is Caldo Verde (page 148). The second is this spicy, ground beef taco meat, which she is crazy about. If I'm in real trouble, I'll make some Cassava Flour Tortillas (page 226), cross my fingers, and hope she finds it in her heart (and belly) to forgive me for whatever it is I don't know I did wrong! Try topping the tacos with Guacamole (page 232) and some finely chopped fresh cilantro and onion, and serve them with lime wedges.

In a small saucepan, combine the stock, ancho chile, and New Mexico chile. Bring to a boil over high heat, remove from the heat, and cover with a lid. Let the chiles soak until soft, about 15 minutes. Stem and seed the chiles and transfer the flesh to a high-speed blender. Add the stock and blend on high until very smooth. Set aside.

In a large sauté pan or Dutch oven, heat the avocado oil over medium-high heat. Working in batches, add the ground beef and cook, breaking up the meat with a wooden spoon as it cooks, until browned, about 12 minutes. Use a slotted spoon to transfer the browned meat to a bowl and repeat to brown the remaining meat.

Discard all but 2 tablespoons of the fat from the pan. Return the pan to medium heat and add the onion and ¼ teaspoon of the salt. Cook, scraping up any browned bits from the bottom of the pan, until the onion is soft and translucent, 3 to 4 minutes. Add the garlic and cook, stirring, for 1 minute. Add the granulated onion, paprika, cumin, oregano, and remaining ½ teaspoon salt and cook, stirring, for 1 minute more.

Add the beef and the pureed chile mixture to the pan and toss to coat. Bring the mixture to a simmer, reduce the heat to low, cover, and cook, stirring occasionally, for at least 30 minutes or up to 1½ hours for a more concentrated flavor. Taste and adjust the salt before serving.

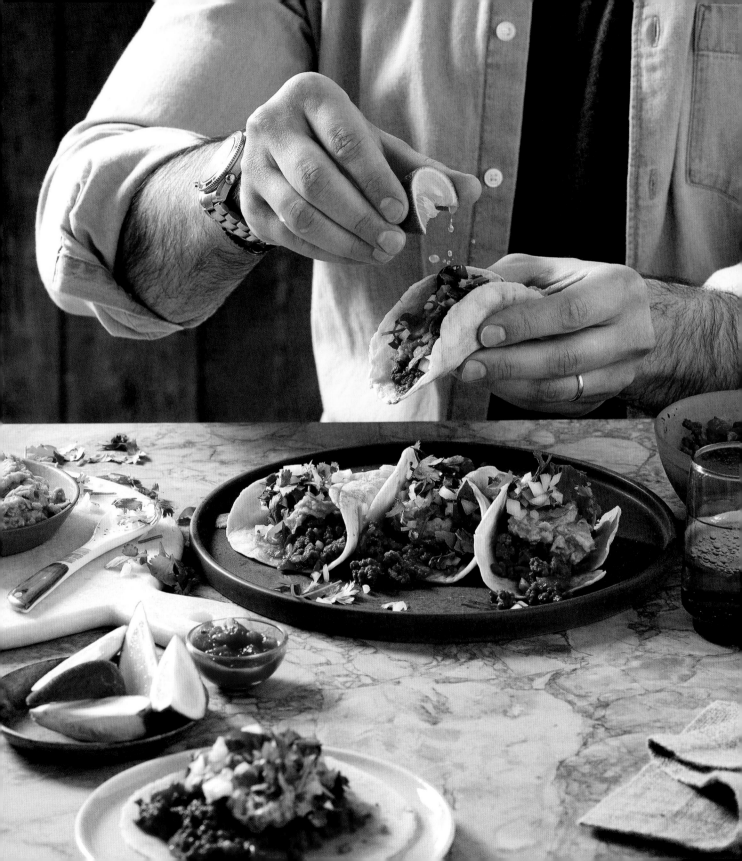

BASIL BEEF

Gluten-Free
Dairy-Free
Whole30
Paleo
Grain-Free
Sugar-Free

Time: 20 minutes

¼ cup coconut aminos

2 garlic cloves, finely chopped

1 teaspoon grated fresh ginger

1 teaspoon arrowroot starch

½ teaspoon fish sauce

1 to 2 tablespoons coconut oil

2 top sirloin medallions (8 ounces total), thinly sliced against the grain

2 carrots, thinly sliced on an angle

2 celery stalks, thinly sliced on an angle

2 scallions, white and green parts separated and thinly sliced on an angle

½ cup raw unsalted cashews

1 fresh Thai bird's-eye chile, finely chopped

1 cup loosely packed fresh basil leaves, coarsely chopped if large

Cauliflower Rice (page 205) or steamed jasmine rice, for serving

Top sirloin medallions are an ideal cut for stir-fries such as this one. They are slightly more expensive than top sirloin steaks, though not by much, but don't have any of the gristle. If unavailable, substitute top sirloin, flank, skirt, or flat iron steak. I wouldn't use a more expensive cut, such as rib eye or tenderloin, for this recipe. Once it gets cooked with the sauce and veggies, you probably won't be able to tell the difference anyway.

You can definitely use my Teriyaki Sauce (page 241) instead of the stir-fry sauce I share here. This is a pared-down version that omits toasted sesame oil, which I sometimes leave out because it tends to dominate the other flavors.

In a mason jar, combine the coconut aminos, garlic, ginger, arrowroot starch, and fish sauce. Seal the jar tightly and shake vigorously until the sauce is completely smooth. Set aside.

In a large wok or cast-iron skillet, melt the coconut oil over high heat. Add the beef and cook, undisturbed, until browned on the bottom, 2 to 3 minutes. Add the carrots, celery, scallion whites, cashews, and Thai chile and cook, stirring frequently, until the vegetables have softened slightly but retain some crunch, 4 to 5 minutes. Pour in the coconut aminos sauce and toss to coat. Cook until the sauce has reduced by one-quarter, about 4 minutes. If you find that the sauce is drying out too quickly, add 1 to 2 tablespoons water as needed.

Remove the pan from the heat and sprinkle in the basil and the scallion greens. Toss to combine and serve immediately over cauliflower rice.

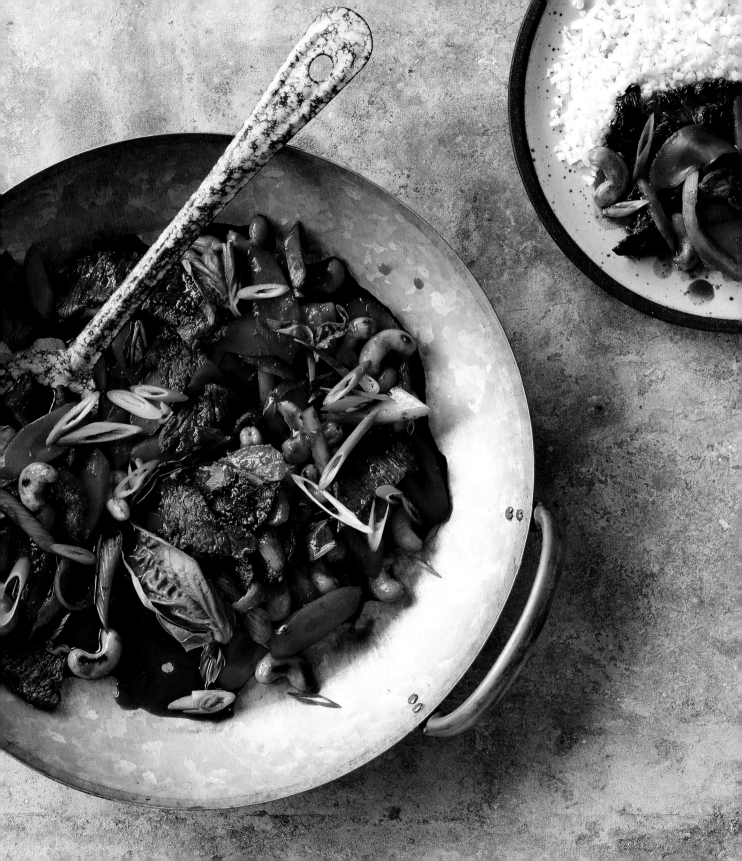

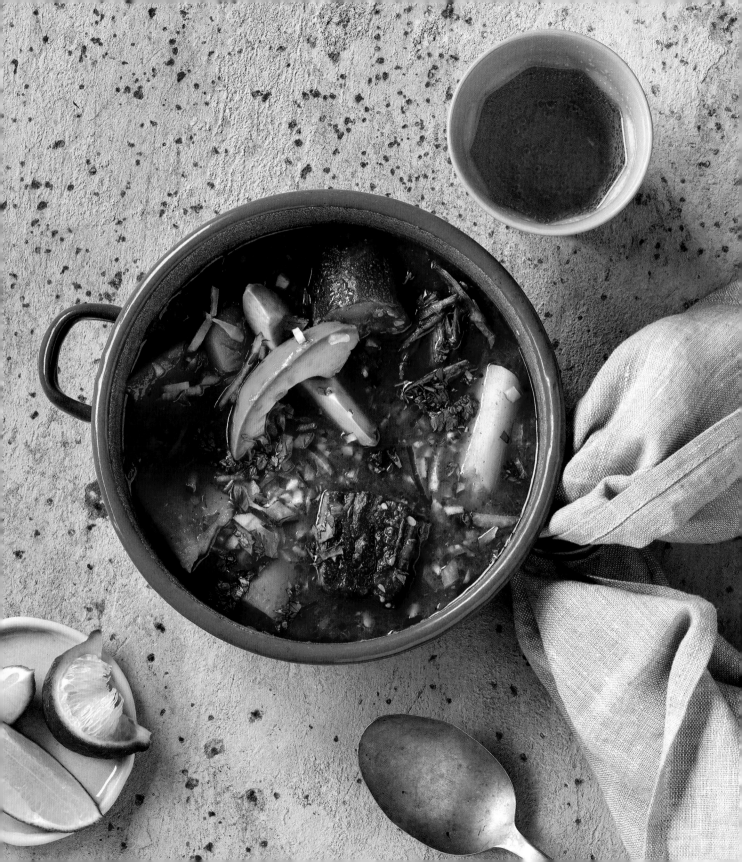

TOMATILLO BEEF SOUP

Similar to my Fauxsole Verde con Pollo (page 66), this Mexican-inspired soup uses tomatillo salsa as a flavorful base. It's loaded with tender, melt-in-your-mouth beef and chunky pieces of potato and zucchini, and topped with thinly sliced red onion, creamy avocado, fresh cilantro, and lime juice. The flavors are incredible, and it's super easy to make, especially if you use a store-bought salsa verde.

MAKE THE SOUP: Lay the beef on a rimmed baking sheet, pat very dry with paper towels, and generously season all sides with salt. Cover with plastic wrap and refrigerate overnight.

An hour before you're ready to cook the beef, remove it from the refrigerator and let it come to room temperature.

In a large Dutch oven, heat the avocado oil over medium-high heat. Pat the beef dry with a paper towel once more and add it to the pan. Cook until the beef is browned on all sides, 12 to 15 minutes total. Transfer the beef to a bowl and set aside.

Add the onion and garlic to the pot and cook, stirring, until beginning to soften, about 2 minutes. Add 4 cups water and cook, stirring with a wooden spoon and scraping up any browned bits from the bottom of the pot, for about 30 seconds. Stir in the salsa verde. Return the beef to the pot, raise the heat to high, and bring the liquid to a boil. Reduce the heat to low, cover, and cook until the beef is tender and easily shredded with two forks, about 2½ hours.

Add the potatoes and zucchini, cover, and cook until the potatoes are fork-tender, about 12 minutes. Taste and adjust the seasoning.

To serve, ladle the soup into individual bowls and garnish with the avocado, red onion, and cilantro. Serve with the lime wedges.

For the Soup:

1½ pounds beef stew meat (such as chuck or short rib), cut into 2-inch cubes

Kosher salt

2 tablespoons avocado oil

1 red onion, diced

4 garlic cloves, smashed and peeled

2 cups salsa verde, store-bought (I like Herdez, which is Whole30 compliant) or homemade (see Fauxsole Verde con Pollo, page 66)

4 Yukon Gold potatoes, peeled and quartered

2 zucchini, cut into 2-inch chunks

For Serving:

2 avocados, sliced into wedges

¼ cup finely chopped red onion

¼ cup finely chopped fresh cilantro leaves

2 limes, cut into wedges

Gluten-Free
Dairy-Free
Whole30
Grain-Free
Sugar-Free

Time: 3¼ hours, plus 12 to 24 hours for marinating

BEEF STROGANOFF

Gluten-Free

Dairy-Free

Whole30

Keto-Friendly

Paleo

Grain-Free

Sugar-Free

Time: 35 minutes

For the Coconut Sour Cream:

1 (13.5-ounce) can full-fat coconut milk, unshaken and refrigerated overnight

Juice of 1 lemon, plus more if needed

For the Stroganoff:

2 tablespoons avocado oil

½ pound beef steak (such as top sirloin medallions, top sirloin, flank, flat iron, or even tenderloin), cut into thin strips

1 tablespoon ghee

1 cup thinly sliced cremini or white button mushrooms

Kosher salt

1 shallot, thinly sliced

3 garlic cloves, thinly sliced

½ cup chicken stock

1 tablespoon whole-grain or Dijon mustard

Freshly ground black pepper

2 tablespoons finely chopped fresh dill, plus more for garnish

Just about everyone has their own spin on beef stroganoff. For my father, that spin was extra garlic, lots of fresh dill, and serving it over potatoes fried in plenty of sunflower oil. He didn't make it often, but when he did, it was a joyous occasion! This version lightens things up by using a coconut "sour cream" in place of regular sour cream, but still delivers all the rich and delicious flavor of my dad's original recipe.

To keep things on the lighter side, try serving the stroganoff over my Oven Fries (page 200) or a bed of fluffy cauliflower grits (see page 162) to soak up all the creamy and delicious sauce.

MAKE THE COCONUT SOUR CREAM: Without shaking the can, carefully open it and spoon the solidified white cream into a medium bowl (save the coconut water left in the can, if you'd like). Add the lemon juice to the coconut cream and whisk until smooth and creamy. Taste and add more lemon juice, if desired. Cover the bowl with plastic wrap and refrigerate until ready to use. (The coconut sour cream will keep in the refrigerator for up to 5 days.)

MAKE THE STROGANOFF: In a large stainless-steel or cast-iron skillet, heat the avocado oil over high heat. Add the steak and cook, undisturbed, until browned on the first side, 2 to 3 minutes. Flip the steak slices and cook for 1 minute, until lightly browned. Transfer the browned steak to a bowl.

Reduce the heat to medium and add the ghee to the pan. When it has melted, add the mushrooms and season with salt. Cook, stirring, until the mushrooms have browned and any moisture they release has evaporated, 4 to 5 minutes. Add the shallot and garlic and cook, scraping up any browned bits from the bottom of the pan, for

recipe continues

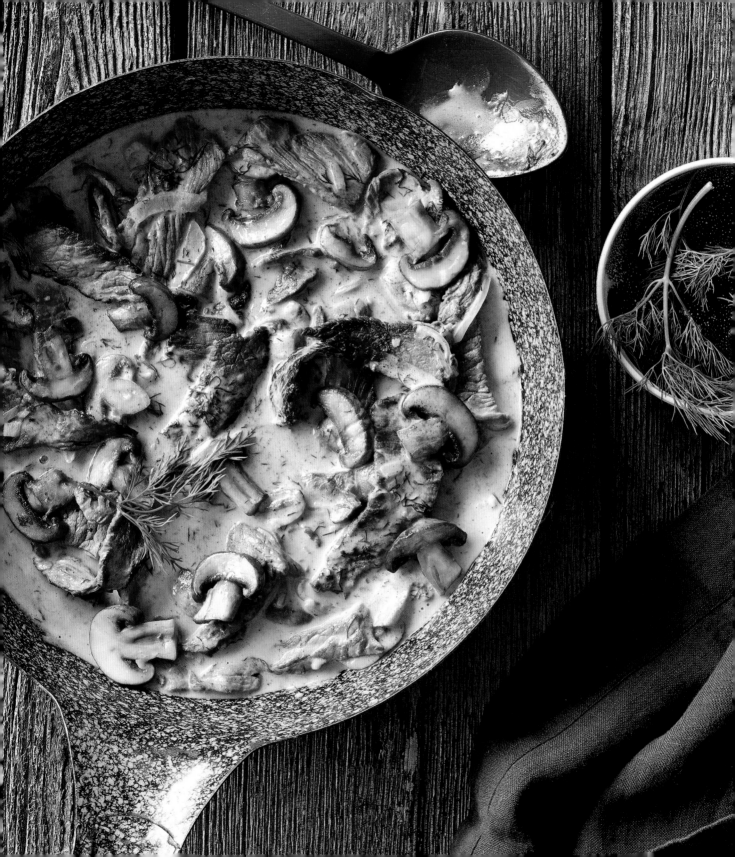

2 to 3 minutes. Pour in the stock and stir, scraping up any stubborn browned bits, and cook until the stock has reduced by one-quarter, about 1 minute.

Add 1 cup of the coconut sour cream (reserve the rest for another use), the mustard, and a pinch of pepper and stir to combine. Gently simmer the sauce for 2 to 3 minutes, reducing the heat if needed to maintain a simmer. Taste and adjust the seasoning as desired. Return the beef to the pan and toss to coat with the sauce. Remove the pan from the heat, sprinkle in the dill, and toss once more to combine. Garnish with more dill and serve immediately.

SWEET POTATOES STUFFED WITH SPICED BEEF, TAHINI, AND PARSLEY SALAD

In the time that it takes to roast the sweet potatoes, you can quickly throw together a delicious and juicy spiced beef, a basic tahini sauce, and a tangy parsley salad. Once assembled, it transforms into a Middle Eastern riff on a loaded baked potato. You may already have all the ingredients on hand. If not, they are readily available. Perhaps the only things you'll have to hunt for are the Aleppo pepper and the sumac. Thankfully, these spices are popping up in more and more specialty stores. Seek out a Middle Eastern grocer in your area first, but if that doesn't pan out, try purchasing the spices online!

Preheat the oven to 400°F.

Rinse the sweet potatoes and scrub them to remove any dirt. Prick them in a few places with a fork and place them on a rimmed baking sheet. Roast for 45 to 50 minutes, until fork-tender.

MAKE THE SPICED BEEF: In a large sauté pan, heat the olive oil over medium-high heat. Add the ground beef and cook, stirring and breaking it up with a spoon as it cooks, until browned, 12 to 15 minutes. Add the onions and cook, stirring, until they are soft and translucent, 6 to 8 minutes. Add the garlic and cook for 2 to 3 minutes. Stir in the coriander, Aleppo pepper, and salt. Pour in ⅔ cup water and scrape up any browned bits from the bottom of the pan. Taste and adjust the seasoning, then cover the pan and remove from the heat.

recipe and ingredients continue

4 sweet potatoes

For the Spiced Beef:

1 tablespoon extra-virgin olive oil

1½ pounds ground beef (80 to 85% lean ground beef is preferred) or ground lamb

2 cups (3 small) diced yellow onions

4 garlic cloves, finely chopped

1 tablespoon ground coriander

1 teaspoon Aleppo pepper

1 teaspoon kosher salt, plus more as needed

For the Parsley Salad:

½ cup fresh parsley leaves, coarsely chopped or torn by hand

1 small red onion, finely sliced

Gluten-Free
Dairy-Free
Whole30
Keto-Friendly
Paleo
Grain-Free
Sugar-Free

Time: 50 minutes

2 tablespoons fresh
lemon juice

2 teaspoons ground
sumac

¼ teaspoon kosher
salt

¼ cup Tahini Sauce
(page 240), for
serving

MAKE THE PARSLEY SALAD: In a medium bowl, toss together the parsley, onion, lemon juice, sumac, and salt. (The parsley salad can be prepared 30 to 60 minutes before serving and stored in the refrigerator—any longer than that, and the parsley will lose its texture.)

To serve, score the top of each sweet potato with a sharp knife and use two spoons to pry the sweet potatoes open. Stuff each potato with a generous serving of the spiced beef. Drizzle with the tahini sauce and top with the parsley salad.

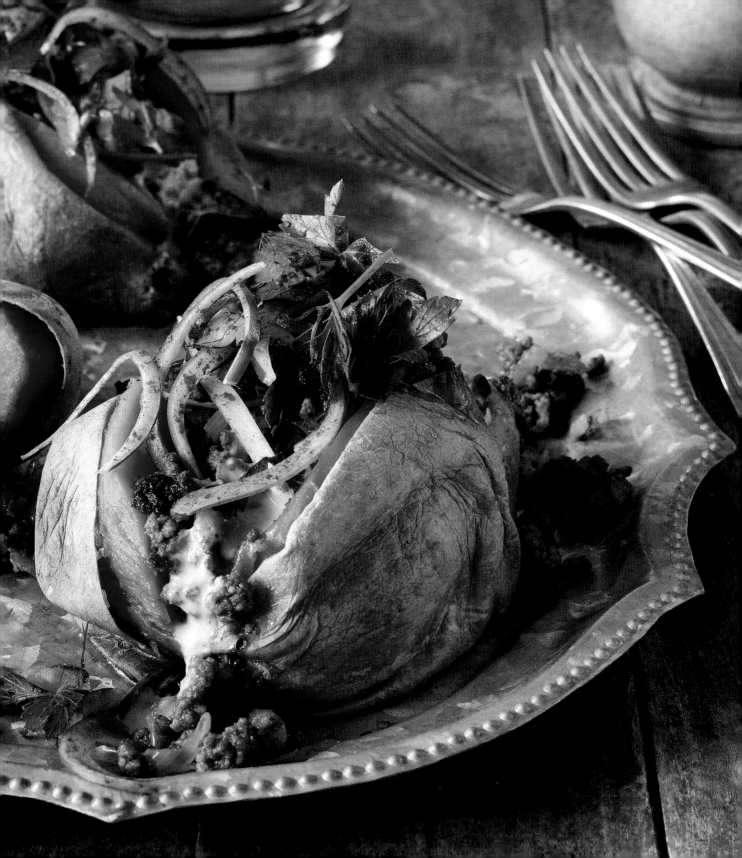

NICU'S MEATBALLS
(CHIFTELUTE MARINATE)

Gluten-Free

Dairy-Free

Whole30

Keto-Friendly

Paleo

Grain-Free

Sugar-Free

Time: 35 minutes

For the Meatballs:

2 pounds ground beef (80 to 85% lean ground beef is preferred)

2 large eggs

½ cup finely chopped fresh parsley leaves

½ cup finely chopped fresh dill

½ red onion, finely chopped

3 garlic cloves, finely chopped

2 teaspoons kosher salt

1 teaspoon baking soda

¼ teaspoon freshly ground black pepper

2 tablespoons extra-virgin olive oil

For the Sauce:

1 tablespoon arrowroot starch

1 (6-ounce) can tomato paste

2 cups chicken stock or water

Kosher salt and freshly ground black pepper

My father-in-law, Nicu, effortlessly threw together a pan of these small meatballs in tomato sauce (*chiftelute marinate*, pronounced *keef-te-loo-tse ma-ree-nah-te*) one night on a family vacation in Romania. Maybe it was the fresh dill, which added an unexpected pop of flavor? Maybe it was the light and airy meatballs themselves? Either way, they were so good that the next day I asked him to make them again, only this time, I wanted to take notes! The only change I made to his original recipe is to use arrowroot starch instead of the white flour he used to thicken the sauce. The result is nearly identical, but with the benefit of being gluten-free.

In Romania, these meatballs are commonly served over a bed of mashed potatoes, which can be made Whole30-compliant if you prepare them without dairy. For a Paleo option, try my Garlicky Mashed Sweet Potatoes (page 199). For something a bit more indulgent, serve them with boiled egg noodles.

MAKE THE MEATBALLS: In a large bowl, combine the ground beef, eggs, parsley, dill, onion, garlic, salt, baking soda, and pepper. Use clean hands to mix until well combined. Test the seasoning by frying a small amount of the mixture in a dry nonstick skillet over medium-high heat. Taste the cooked portion and season the raw mixture with salt and pepper, as needed. Lightly wet your hands and form the mixture into equal-size meatballs slightly larger than golf balls and place on a baking sheet or large plate.

In a large nonstick skillet, heat the olive oil over medium-high heat. Working in batches, add the meatballs and cook until browned on all sides and fully cooked through, 15 to 17 minutes total. Transfer the cooked meatballs to a baking sheet and tent with aluminum foil to keep warm. Repeat to cook the remaining meatballs. Discard any dark brown bits left the pan and pour off all but 2 tablespoons of the rendered fat from the pan.

MAKE THE SAUCE: Return the pan to the stove and heat the reserved fat over medium heat. Add the arrowroot starch and cook, stirring continuously with a wooden spoon, for 1 minute. Add the tomato paste and stock and season with salt and pepper. Cook, stirring often, until thickened, 3 to 4 minutes. Add the garlic and cook until fragrant, about 2 minutes. If the sauce becomes too thick, stir in 1 to 2 tablespoons water to loosen it. Add the parsley and dill, taste, and adjust the seasoning, if needed.

Remove the pan from the heat, add the meatballs to the sauce, and toss to coat. Serve immediately.

3 garlic cloves, finely sliced

1 tablespoon finely chopped fresh parsley leaves

1 tablespoon finely chopped fresh dill

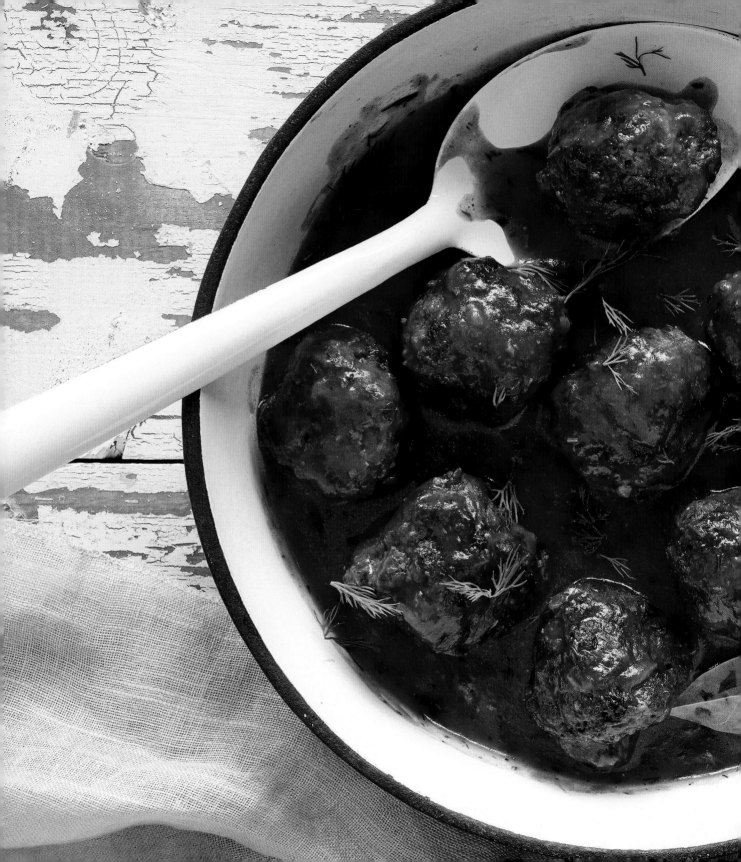

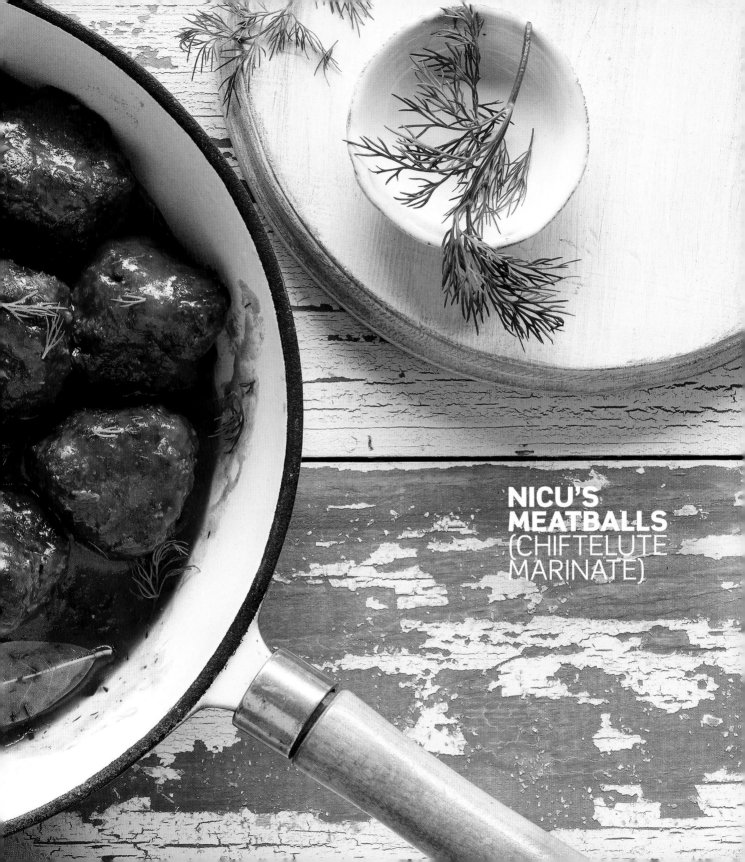

NICU'S MEATBALLS
(CHIFTELUTE MARINATE)

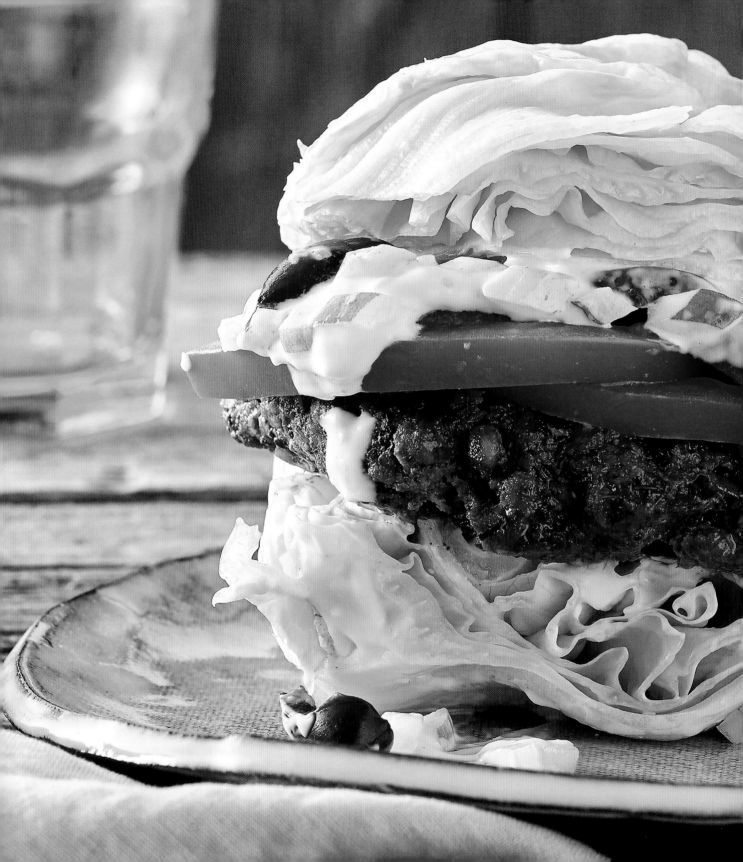

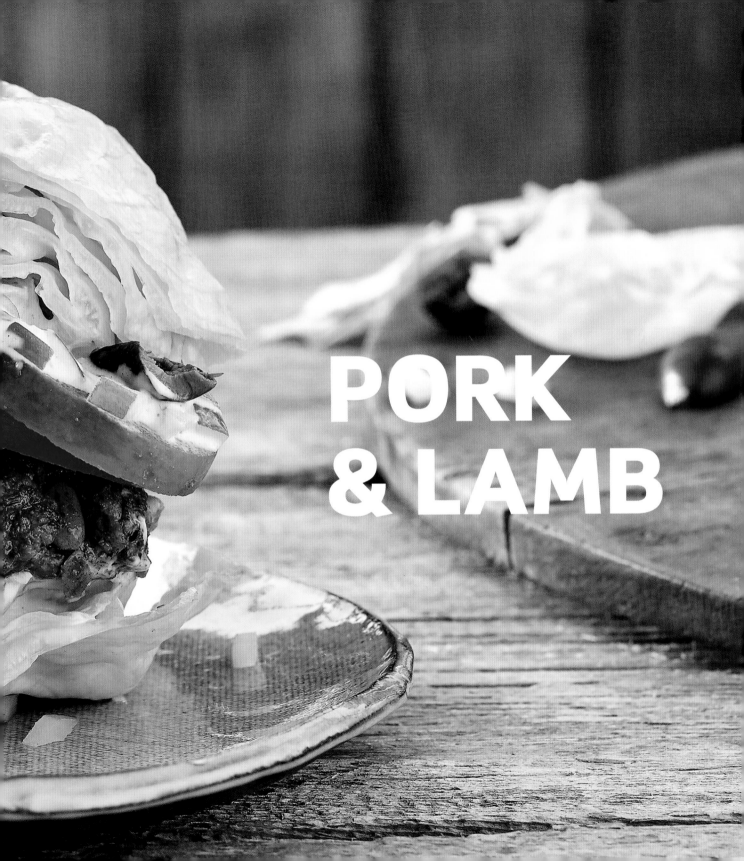

PORK & LAMB

GRILLED CHIMICHURRI PORK CHOPS

Gluten-Free

Dairy-Free

Whole30

Keto-Friendly

Paleo

Grain-Free

Sugar-Free

Time: 25 minutes,
plus at least
4 hours of
marinating

4 (10-ounce)
center-cut bone-in
pork chops, about
1½ inches thick

Kosher salt and
freshly ground black
pepper

1 cup Cha Cha
Chimichurri
(page 235)

As I mention on page 235, my Cha Cha Chimichurri isn't just great as a sauce—it also makes a killer marinade! Try it with some beautiful center-cut bone-in pork chops for an easy and delicious protein option. If you find yourself with leftovers, which is doubtful, try slicing the cold chops paper-thin and draping them over my Fauxttoush salad (page 8) for a delicious lunch the next day.

Generously season both sides of each pork chop with salt and pepper. Transfer the chops to a large zip-top plastic bag and add half the chimichurri. Massage the pork chops to coat with the chimichurri, then squeeze as much air out of the bag as possible and seal. Set on a rimmed baking sheet and refrigerate for at least 4 hours or up to overnight.

Heat a grill to medium-high or heat a grill pan over medium-high heat. Grill the pork chops, without moving them, until grill marks form, about 4 minutes. Rotate the chops 90 degrees and cook until grill marks form, about 2 minutes. Flip the chops and repeat, until the chops reach your desired doneness (between 145° and 160°F).

Let the pork chops rest for 5 minutes before serving with the remaining chimichurri.

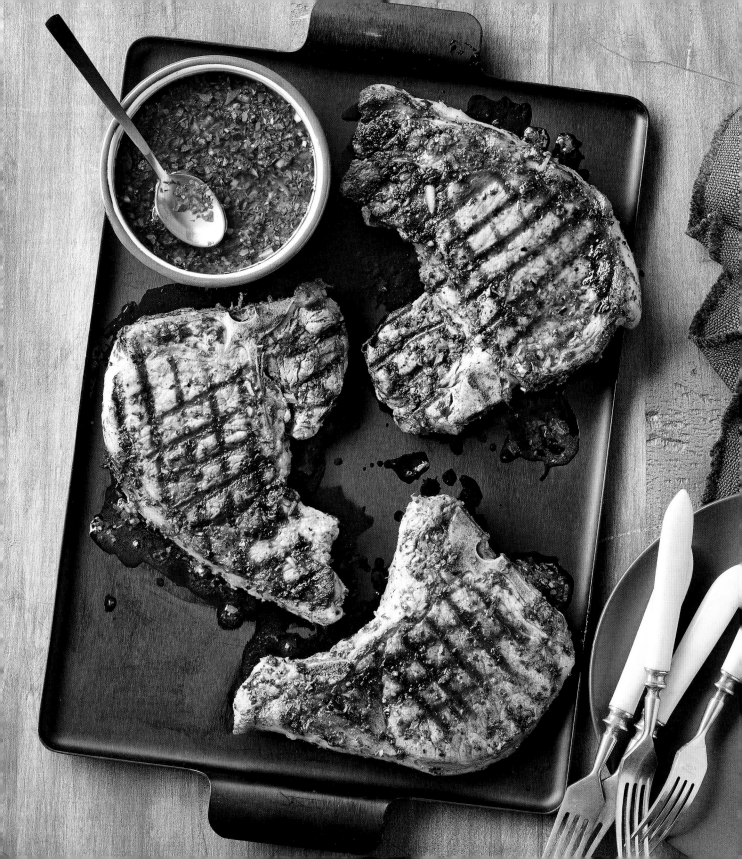

MOROCCAN LAMB STEW
WITH APRICOTS AND CHICKPEAS

Gluten-Free

Dairy-Free

Grain-Free

Sugar-Free

Time: 2¾ hours

2 tablespoons avocado oil

2 pounds lamb stew meat, cut into 2-inch cubes

1 large yellow onion, diced

6 small carrots (about 1 pound), cut into rounds

Kosher salt

4 garlic cloves, coarsely chopped

1 teaspoon ground ginger

1 teaspoon ground cumin

½ teaspoon ground cinnamon

½ teaspoon cayenne pepper

1 (13.5-ounce) can diced tomatoes, with their juices

½ cup dried apricots

4 cups chicken stock, as needed

1 (15.5-ounce) can chickpeas, drained and rinsed

Subtle notes of earthy spices like ginger and cinnamon are balanced by the sweetness of apricots in this delicious lamb stew. The starchy chickpeas are neither Paleo nor Whole30, but they are something I often find myself craving. Personally, I can tolerate them in moderation and love to incorporate them into stews like this one or puree them into homemade Creamy Hummus (page 222). They're a nice break from potatoes, very filling, and super affordable. If you'd like to keep things Whole30, replace the chickpeas with diced potato (make it diced sweet potato for a Paleo version).

In a large Dutch oven or heavy-bottomed pot, heat the avocado oil over medium-high heat. Working in batches, add the lamb and cook until browned on all sides, about 15 minutes total. Transfer the browned meat to a plate and repeat to cook the remaining lamb.

Add the onion and carrots to the pot and season with a pinch of salt. Cook, stirring often, until the vegetables have softened, 8 to 10 minutes. Use your spoon to scrape up any browned bits from the bottom of the pot; if they don't want to budge, add 1 to 2 tablespoons water. Add the garlic and cook, stirring, for 1 minute. Add the ginger, cumin, cinnamon, and cayenne and cook, stirring, just until the spices are fragrant, about 1 minute.

Return the lamb to the pot and add the tomatoes with their liquid and the apricots. Stir to combine. Pour in just enough stock to barely cover the meat (you may not need all 4 cups). Bring to a steady simmer, then reduce the heat to low, cover, and cook, stirring occasionally, until the lamb is very tender, 1½ to 2 hours.

Stir in the chickpeas and cook for 10 minutes. Taste and season with more salt as desired.

Ladle the stew into individual bowls, garnish with the parsley and toasted almonds, and serve.

¼ cup loosely packed fresh parsley leaves, finely chopped, for garnish

¼ cup slivered toasted almonds, for garnish

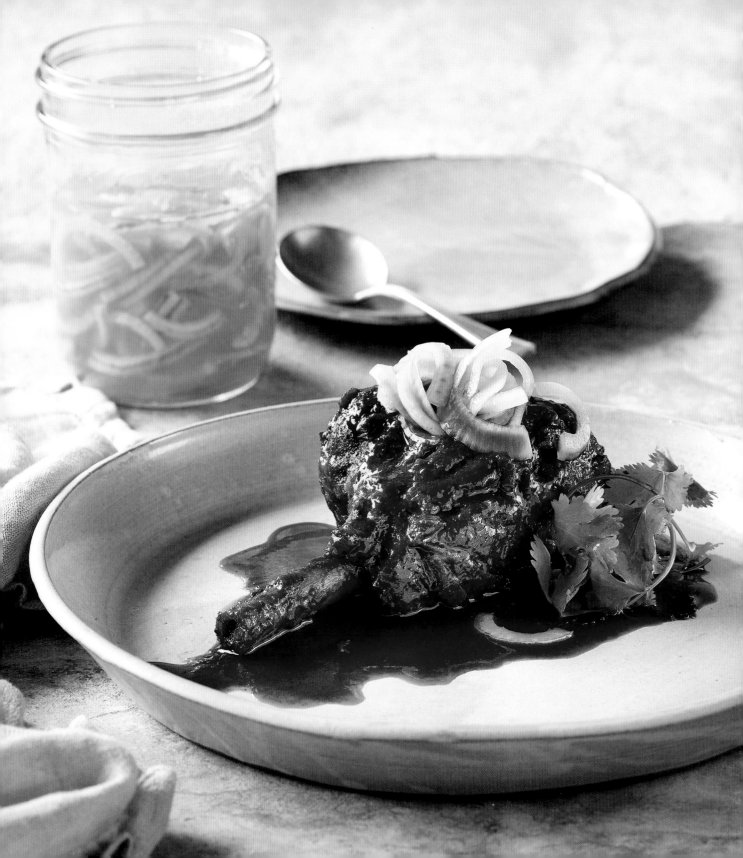

ANCHO-BRAISED LAMB SHANKS
WITH QUICK-PICKLED ONIONS

This Mexican-inspired braised lamb shank is absolutely bursting with flavor. The secret is to use dried whole chiles, which are thankfully becoming more and more available in grocery stores. I use a combination of ancho and guajillo chiles, but you should feel free to experiment with other varieties, like morita (smoked jalapeño), cascabel, pasilla, or chiles de árbol, to name a few.

To cut through the rich, fatty lamb and balance the earthy spiciness in the braising liquid, I top the shanks with my quick-pickled red onions. They're bright and acidic, and they look beautiful on the plate. Try serving the lamb shanks with Cauliflower Rice (page 205), or steamed rice, if you're living your Food Freedom, and a side salad.

Pat the lamb shanks dry with paper towels and liberally season all sides with salt. Set aside at room temperature for 1 hour or cover and refrigerate for up to 24 hours. If refrigerating the lamb shanks, let them come to room temperature before cooking.

In a large Dutch oven, toast the ancho and guajillo chiles over medium-low heat, flipping them occasionally, until slightly softened, about 4 minutes.

In a 2-quart saucepan, bring the stock to a boil over high heat. Add the toasted chiles to the stock. Cover with a tight-fitting lid, remove the pot from the heat, and let the chiles soak for 15 minutes.

Remove the chiles, reserving the stock, and place them on a cutting board. Stem and seed them and transfer the flesh and skin to

recipe continues

---

4 (8-ounce) lamb shanks

Kosher salt

3 dried whole ancho chiles

1 dried whole guajillo chile

2 cups beef stock or chicken stock

2 tablespoons avocado oil

1 large yellow onion, thinly sliced

4 garlic cloves, coarsely chopped

1 teaspoon smoked Spanish paprika

1 teaspoon hot paprika

1 teaspoon ground coriander

1 teaspoon ground cumin

1 teaspoon dried oregano

Quick-Pickled Red Onions (see page 143), for serving

Gluten-Free

Dairy-Free

Whole30

Keto-Friendly

Paleo

Grain-Free

Sugar-Free

Time: 3 hours, plus 1 hour of resting

PORK & LAMB

a high-speed blender. Add the stock and blend on high speed until completely smooth. Set aside.

Heat the same Dutch oven over medium heat for at least 5 minutes. Increase the heat to medium-high and add the avocado oil. Heat the oil until it's shimmering, then add the lamb shanks in batches and brown on all sides, about 15 minutes total. Transfer the lamb to a bowl and set aside.

Add the sliced onion to the pot, season with salt, and cook, stirring, until slightly softened, 3 to 4 minutes. Add the garlic and cook, stirring, for 1 minute. Stir in the smoked paprika, hot paprika, coriander, cumin, and oregano and toss to coat the onion and garlic. Toast the mixture for 1 minute, then stir in the pureed chile mixture. Return the lamb to the pot and stir to coat it in the sauce. Cover, reduce the heat to low, and cook until the meat is falling off the bone, 1½ to 2 hours.

Transfer the lamb shanks to a plate and set aside. Place a fine-mesh sieve over a large bowl and strain the sauce from the pot. Discard the solids and let the sauce sit, undisturbed, for 5 minutes so the fat rises to the top. Using a spoon, remove as much fat from the surface of the sauce as possible. Return the sauce to the pot and cook over medium heat until reduced by about one-quarter, about 8 minutes.

Return the lamb shanks to the pot and stir to coat them in the sauce. Serve the lamb and sauce topped with quick-pickled red onions.

CURRY LAMB AND POTATOES

I tested a lot of recipes while writing this book, and I can honestly say that none of them were as pleasantly surprising as this lamb and potato curry. For something so simple and with so few ingredients, it is unbelievably delicious.

My only word of caution is that certain brands of coconut milk have a tendency to separate when cooking. There are three things I do to prevent this. The first is I buy a brand of full-fat coconut milk that I've used before and know won't separate. My personal favorites are Aroy-D coconut milk and Savoy coconut cream. Second, if the coconut milk has already separated in the can, I use an immersion blender to re-emulsify it. Third, I find that it helps to add the coconut milk to the pot in stages. I do this in halves, with the first half going in to deglaze the pot after I've sautéed the onions and spices. Not only will this help to temper the coconut milk and prevent curdling, but it also allows me to see any browned bits that need to be lifted off the bottom of the pot with a wooden spoon.

Pat the lamb dry with paper towels and liberally season all sides with salt.

In a large Dutch oven, melt the coconut oil over medium-low heat. Add the lamb and brown on all sides, 12 to 15 minutes total; work in batches if needed so as not to crowd the pan. Transfer the browned meat to a bowl and set aside.

Add the onion, garlic, and a pinch of salt to the pot. Cook, scraping up any browned bits from the bottom of the pot, until the onion is slightly soft, 4 to 5 minutes. Add the curry powder, stir to coat the onion, and cook for another minute.

2 pounds lamb stew meat, cut into 2-inch cubes

Kosher salt

2 tablespoons coconut oil

1 large yellow onion, sliced

4 garlic cloves, coarsely chopped

1 tablespoon curry powder

1 (14-ounce) can full-fat coconut milk

2 pounds Yukon Gold potatoes, peeled and quartered

2 bay leaves

1 fresh red chile, such as Anaheim or finger, thinly sliced

¼ cup fresh cilantro leaves, for garnish

Gluten-Free

Dairy-Free

Whole30

Keto-Friendly

Paleo

Grain-Free

Sugar-Free

Time: 2 hours

recipe continues

Add about half the coconut milk and again scrape up any browned bits from the bottom of the pot. Once you can see that there are no more stuck-on brown bits, add the remaining coconut milk, the browned lamb, potatoes, bay leaves, and chile. Pour in enough water to nearly cover the meat and potatoes. Stir everything to combine. Bring to a boil, then reduce the heat to low, cover, and cook until the lamb is tender, about 1½ hours. Taste and adjust the seasoning as desired.

Ladle into individual serving bowls, garnish with the cilantro leaves, and serve.

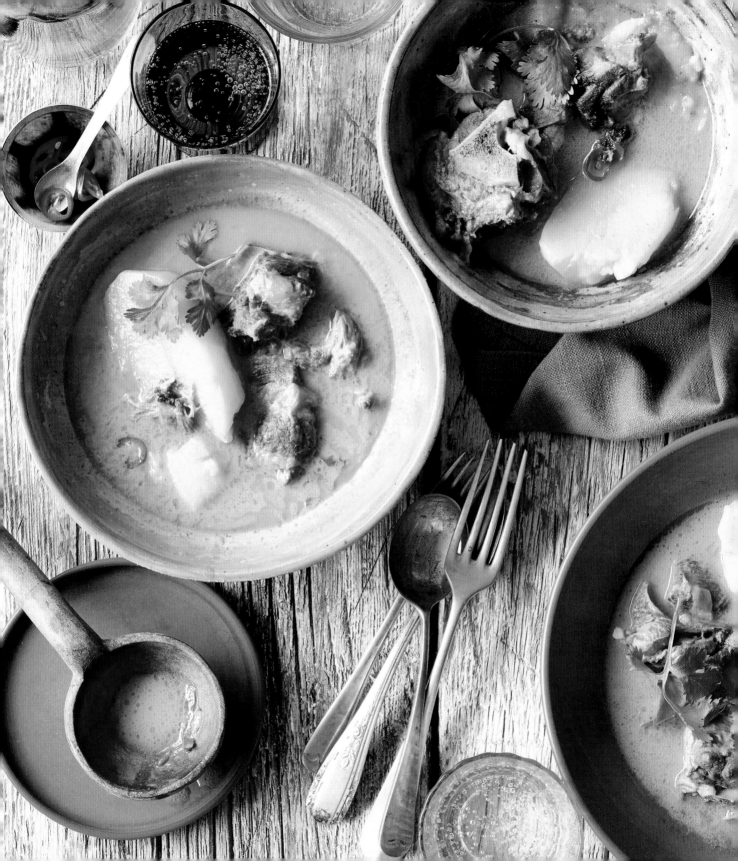

JERK RIBS

Gluten-Free
Dairy-Free
Whole30
Keto-Friendly
Paleo
Grain-Free
Sugar-Free

Time: 4 hours,
plus at least
4 hours of
marinating

2 (1½-pound) racks of
pork back or side ribs

1 cup Jerk Rub
(page 257)

Use my versatile Jerk Rub (page 257) to infuse these ribs with
a tremendous amount of flavor. Just like my Roast Short Ribs
(page 92), these spicy pork ribs are roasted low and slow with a
splash of water until they're falling off the bone and super juicy. Try
serving them with some Sweet Plantains (Maduros) (page 210) and
Caraway Cabbage Coleslaw (page 2).

On a cutting board, place the ribs meat-side down and use a paring
knife to pull up an edge of the translucent membrane. Grab hold of
the membrane with a paper towel and slowly peel it back until you
have removed it completely. Discard the membrane.

Cut the ribs in half, put them in a large zip-top plastic bag, and pour
in the Jerk Rub. Massage to coat, squeeze as much air out of the bag
as possible, and seal the bag. Set it on a rimmed baking sheet and
refrigerate for 4 to 24 hours.

Preheat the oven to 275°F. Line a roasting pan with parchment paper.

Remove the ribs from the marinade and let any excess marinade
drip off (discard the bag). Place the ribs bone-side down in the prepared roasting pan. Add ½ cup water to the bottom of the pan and
wrap the pan tightly in aluminum foil. Place the pan on the lowest
rack of the oven and bake for 4 hours, or until the meat is falling off
the bone. Serve immediately.

COCHINITA PIBIL

Cochinita pibil, or *puerco pibil*, is a Yucatán-style slow-roasted pork. Though recipes differ, it is commonly made by first marinating a whole suckling pig in a mixture of achiote (or annatto) seeds, cloves, allspice, oregano, sour orange, garlic, and other spices or herbs. The pig is then wrapped in banana leaves, placed into a pit lined with hot stones, and slowly cooked until the meat is falling off the bone.

Aside from the ingredients, which we'll get to in a second, the biggest impact on the taste of your *cochinita pibil* is the method you use to cook it. Dry heat, smoke, and steam will each bring something different to the table, pun intended. And yes, I know, none of these can truly be called *cochinita pibil* because they aren't cooked in a *pib* (the Mayan word for a cooking pit). But let's just go with it.

Depending on its thickness, a bone-in pork shoulder will need to cook for at least 4 hours on high heat or between 7 and 8 hours on low heat. If the pork shoulder is boneless, you can probably shave an hour off the low-heat cooking time. The only thing I'm not crazy about with the slow cooker is the lack of some dry heat, which changes the way the banana leaves taste. When they're steamed, as they are in the slow cooker, I find that their intense flavor is amplified. Personally, if I'm using a slow cooker for this dish, I omit the banana leaves altogether because I don't want their flavor overpowering the subtlety of the pork and marinade.

MAKE THE PORK SHOULDER: In a blender, combine the achiote paste, orange juice, and lime juice and blend until smooth.

Dry the pork shoulder thoroughly with paper towels. Liberally season all sides of the pork with salt and place it in a large bowl or large zip-top plastic bag set on a rimmed baking sheet (to catch any juices). Pour in the marinade. Massage the marinade all over the pork to coat. Cover (or seal the bag) and refrigerate for at least 4 hours or up to 24 hours.

For the Pork Shoulder:

¼ cup achiote paste, such as El Yucateco

½ cup fresh orange juice

¼ cup fresh lime juice

1 (3½-pound) pork shoulder, preferably bone-in

Kosher salt

2 large banana leaves, rinsed and wiped clean (optional)

For the Quick-Pickled Red Onions:

¼ cup apple cider vinegar

1 tablespoon agave nectar (omit for Whole30)

¼ teaspoon kosher salt

1 large red onion, thinly sliced

For Serving:

1 green cabbage, thinly sliced

2 limes, cut into wedges

½ cup fresh cilantro leaves

Gluten-Free

Dairy-Free

Paleo

Grain-Free

Sugar-Free

Time: 4 to 8 hours, depending on cooking method, plus at least 4 hours of marinating

Slow cooker method: 8 hours, plus 4 hours of marinating

Oven method: 4 hours, plus 4 hours of marinating

recipe continues

PORK & LAMB

SLOW COOKER METHOD: Remove the pork from the marinade, letting any excess drip off (discard the excess marinade). Place the pork in a slow cooker. Cover and cook on Low for 7 to 8 hours or on High for at least 4 hours, until the meat is falling off the bone.

OVEN METHOD: Preheat the oven to 300°F. Line a 4-inch-deep roasting pan with one banana leaf.

Remove the pork from the marinade, letting any excess drip off (discard the excess marinade). Place the pork in the center of the pan and top it with the second banana leaf; wrap it tightly. Add ½ cup water to the bottom of the pan, cover the pan with aluminum foil, and bake for 3½ to 4 hours, until the meat is falling off the bone.

MAKE THE QUICK-PICKLED RED ONIONS: In a small saucepan, combine the vinegar, agave nectar, salt, and ½ cup water. Bring to a gentle simmer over medium-high heat and cook, stirring often, until the agave and salt have dissolved, 2 to 3 minutes. Pack the sliced onion into a pint-size mason jar and pour in the hot pickling liquid. Let stand at room temperature for at least 30 minutes before serving, or until completely cooled before refrigerating. (The onions will keep, covered, in the refrigerator for up to 2 weeks.)

TO SERVE: Transfer the cooked pork to a large bowl and shred the meat with two forks. Transfer all the juices from the slow cooker or roasting pan to a jar or bowl to reserve for serving. Spoon some of the juices over the pork. Serve with the pickled onions, shredded cabbage, lime wedges, cilantro, and the reserved cooking juices.

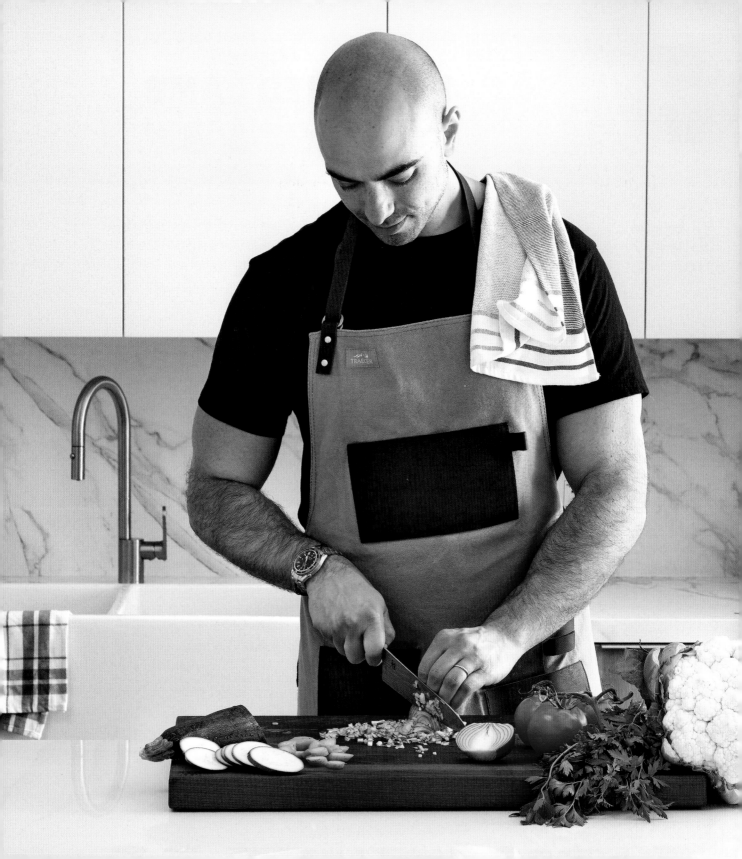

PAN-FRIED LAMB CHOPS WITH PAPA'S HERBY KETCHUP

Gluten-Free

Dairy-Free

Whole30

Keto-Friendly

Paleo

Grain-Free

Sugar-Free

Time: 20 minutes

1½ pounds lamb rib or loin chops

2 tablespoons avocado oil

Kosher salt and freshly ground black pepper

1 cup Papa's Herby Ketchup (page 239)

One of the meals I associate most with my childhood is pan-fried lamb chops. To say that my father loves lamb is an understatement (which is a bit strange, because he doesn't eat other red meat). Maybe once a week, he'd come home from work with a pack of lamb chops that he'd pick up from the butcher. He'd unwrap the pink butcher paper and quickly season the chops with salt and pepper before throwing them into a screaming-hot pan with a bit of oil. Before long, the kitchen would be completely filled with smoke because there was no range vent in my parents' kitchen. The smoke would creep under the kitchen door and travel upstairs to our bedrooms. Along with it came the aroma of lamb fat getting crispy. I'd immediately run downstairs to see if I could manage to grab one of the chops he'd already finished frying. My brother often beat me to the chase.

Without fail, my father served the lamb chops with canned peas and corn, maybe some chopped tomatoes and cucumbers if we had them, and his famous herby ketchup. This tomato-based sauce is very pungent, especially for the uninitiated, but boy, oh boy, is it tasty!

Rub the lamb chops all over with the avocado oil and liberally season both sides with salt and pepper.

Heat a 12-inch cast-iron skillet over medium heat for at least 5 minutes. Increase the heat to medium-high, add the lamb chops, and cook, undisturbed, until browned on the bottom, 4 to 5 minutes. Flip and cook on the second side to your desired doneness (145°F for medium-rare, which is what I recommend), 4 to 5 minutes.

Serve the chops with the herby ketchup.

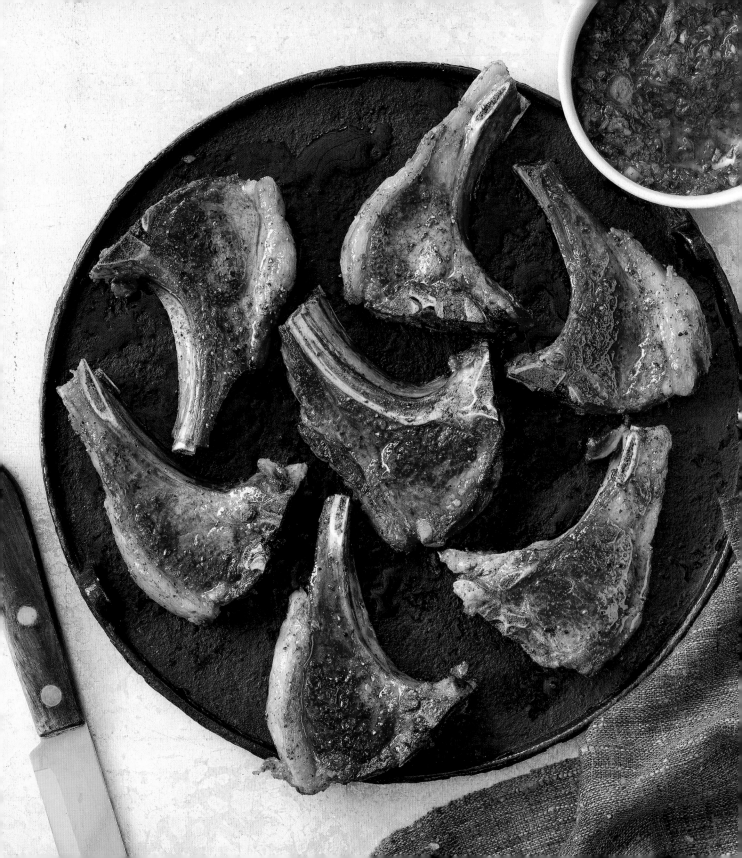

CALDO VERDE

Gluten-Free
Dairy-Free
Whole30
Paleo
Grain-Free
Sugar-Free

Time: 60 minutes

- 2 tablespoons extra-virgin olive oil
- 1 large white onion, sliced or coarsely chopped
- Kosher salt
- 3 garlic cloves, smashed and peeled
- 1 tablespoon smoked Spanish paprika
- 1 teaspoon cayenne pepper (optional)
- 4 cups chicken stock
- 3 Japanese yams or yellow potatoes, peeled and cut into 2-inch cubes
- ½ pound cured (Spanish) chorizo, sliced into thin discs
- 1 large bunch collard greens, leaves stemmed and sliced into thin ribbons

This is my wife's absolute favorite dish and my get-out-of-jail-free card. If I leave town for a few days on business, I make her a big pot. If I'm in the doghouse for something I did wrong, I make her a big pot. If I forget her birthday—not that I ever have or ever will!—I'll make her a big pot. No matter the gravity of the situation, *caldo verde* (a Portuguese dish that translates as "green soup") makes things right. Except for that one time I accidentally burned a hole in her favorite blouse with the iron. There was no coming back from that one.

In a large Dutch oven or heavy-bottomed pot, heat the olive oil over medium-high heat. Add the onion and season with salt. Cook, stirring, until the onion is soft and translucent, 10 to 12 minutes. Add the garlic and cook, stirring, until tender and fragrant but not browned, 1 to 2 minutes. Add the paprika and cayenne (if using) and cook, stirring continuously to avoid burning the spices, for just 1 minute.

Stir in the stock, yams, and 4 cups water. Increase the heat to high and bring the liquid to a gentle boil. Cover the pot with the lid ajar and cook until the yams are fork-tender, 10 to 12 minutes.

Remove the pot from the heat and, using an immersion blender, blend the soup directly in the pot until smooth. (Alternatively, let the soup cool briefly, then carefully ladle it into a blender and blend until smooth; return the blended soup to the pot.) Increase the heat to maintain a simmer and add the chorizo and collards. Cook until the chorizo is softened slightly and the collards have significantly wilted and reduced in volume, about 10 minutes.

Taste and adjust the seasoning. Ladle into individual bowls and serve.

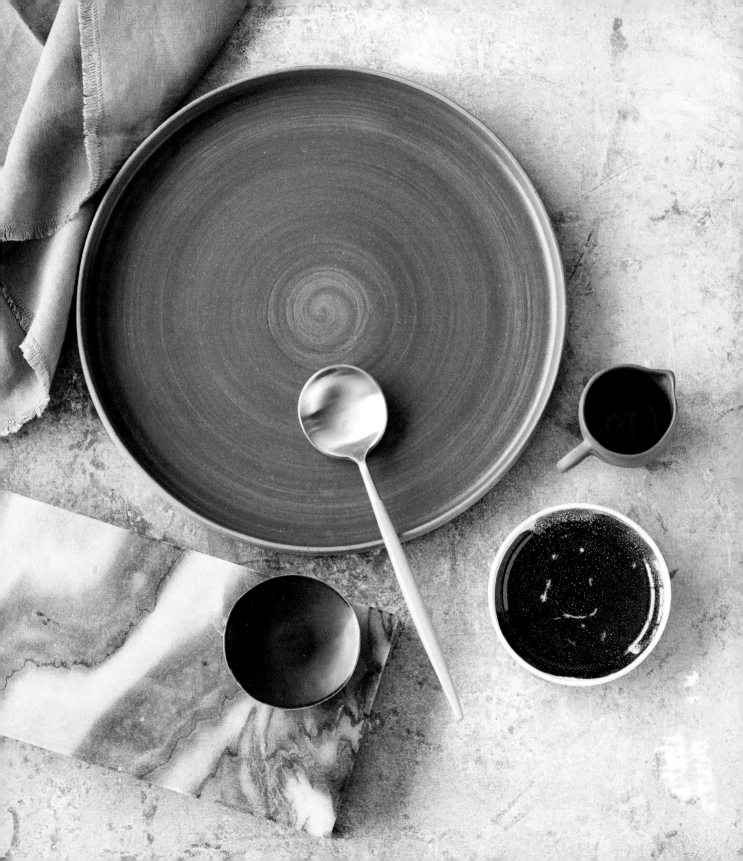

SLOW COOKER MOJO PORK

Gluten-Free
Dairy-Free
Whole30
Paleo
Grain-Free
Sugar-Free

Time: 3 to 8 hours, depending on cooking method, plus 24 hours of marinating

Slow cooker method: 8 hours, plus 24 hours of marinating

Oven method: 4¼ hours, plus 24 hours of marinating

½ cup fresh orange juice

½ cup fresh lime juice

¼ cup extra-virgin olive oil

4 garlic cloves, coarsely chopped

1 tablespoon ground coriander

1 teaspoon dried oregano

1 (3- to 4-pound) bone-in pork shoulder

Kosher salt and freshly ground black pepper

¼ cup loosely packed fresh cilantro leaves, finely chopped

8 fresh mint leaves, finely chopped

Inspired by a delicious roast pork at La Cubana in Toronto, one of my favorite restaurants in the city, this *mojo* pork is fall-off-the-bone tender, bursting with flavor, and, thanks to the slow cooker, incredibly easy to prepare. It's perfect for a Sunday lunch, and any leftovers can be eaten throughout the week. Try it with some fried eggs and Twice-Fried Plantains (page 218) or Sweet Plantains (Maduros) (page 210) for the most incredible breakfast or lunch!

The marinade is identical to the one in my Mojo Loco Chicken Wings (page 46). I told you it was versatile! The key difference here is that I don't blend the mojo to make a sauce after using it as a marinade. Instead, I like to use the rendered cooking juices as a kind of broth, and add fresh cilantro and mint leaves to it after cooking. The sweet-and-sour juices drip down and coat all the shredded bits of meat, and the fresh herbs add color, flavor, and texture.

In a blender or food processor, combine the orange juice, lime juice, olive oil, garlic, coriander, and oregano and blend until completely smooth.

Using a fork, poke the pork shoulder all over. Liberally season all sides of the meat with salt and pepper. Put the pork in a large zip-top plastic bag set on a rimmed baking sheet (to catch any juices). Pour in the marinade. Massage the pork to coat with the marinade, squeeze as much air out of the bag as possible, and seal the bag. Refrigerate the pork overnight.

SLOW COOKER METHOD: Transfer the pork and all of the marinade to a slow cooker. Cover and cook on Low for 6 to 8 hours or on High for 3 to 4 hours, until the meat is falling off the bone.

OVEN METHOD: Preheat the oven to 300°F.

Transfer the pork and all of the marinade to a 4-inch-deep roasting pan, cover the pan with aluminum foil, and roast for 3½ to 4 hours, until the meat is falling off the bone.

TO SERVE: Transfer the pork to a bowl and let cool for 10 to 15 minutes, then use two forks to shred the meat.

If desired, set the oven to broil. Transfer the shredded pork to an oven-safe dish and broil in the top third of the oven for 3 to 4 minutes, until crispy.

Transfer all of the rendered juices from the slow cooker or roasting pan to a bowl. Let the juices sit, undisturbed, for 5 minutes so the fat rises to the top. Using a spoon, remove as much fat from the surface of the liquid as possible.

Stir the cilantro and mint into the rendered juices and serve as a sauce for the pork.

POMEGRANATE BRAISED LAMB SHANKS

Gluten-Free

Dairy-Free

Whole30

Paleo

Grain-Free

Time: 2¾ hours, plus 1 hour of marinating

4 (8-ounce) lamb shanks

3 tablespoons avocado oil

1 tablespoon kosher salt

1 tablespoon ground coriander

2 teaspoons ground cumin

½ teaspoon ground cinnamon

2 cups beef stock

2 tablespoons no-sugar-added pomegranate molasses

1 tablespoon arrowroot starch

¼ cup unsalted slivered almonds, toasted, for garnish

2 tablespoons finely chopped fresh parsley leaves, for garnish

Lamb shanks are one of my favorite cuts of meat. They're relatively affordable, incredibly flavorful, and very easy to cook. Here I spice them up with earthy Middle Eastern flavors and make a sauce with pomegranate molasses. This thick syrup is sweet, tangy, and slightly sour and pairs beautifully with the rich, fatty lamb.

It may be a bit of a challenge to find pomegranate molasses that is free of added sugars, but it's worth the effort. Try sourcing some from a Middle Eastern grocer first. If that fails, continue your search online.

Drizzle the lamb shanks with 1 tablespoon of the avocado oil and season all sides with the salt, coriander, cumin, and cinnamon. Cover and set aside at room temperature for 1 hour or refrigerate for up to 24 hours. If you refrigerate the lamb, let it come to room temperature for 1 hour before cooking.

Heat a large Dutch oven over medium heat for at least 5 minutes. Increase the heat to medium-high and add the remaining 2 tablespoons avocado oil, heating until it shimmers. Add the lamb shanks in batches and brown on all sides, 12 to 15 minutes total. Pour in the stock and use a wooden spoon to scrape up any browned bits from the bottom of the pot. Stir in the pomegranate molasses and bring the liquid to a steady simmer. Reduce the heat to low, cover, and cook until the lamb is falling off the bone, 1½ to 2 hours.

Carefully transfer the lamb to a plate and set aside. Pour the cooking juices into a bowl. Let it sit for 5 minutes and then use a large spoon or ladle to skim off as much fat as possible. Return the juices to the

recipe continues

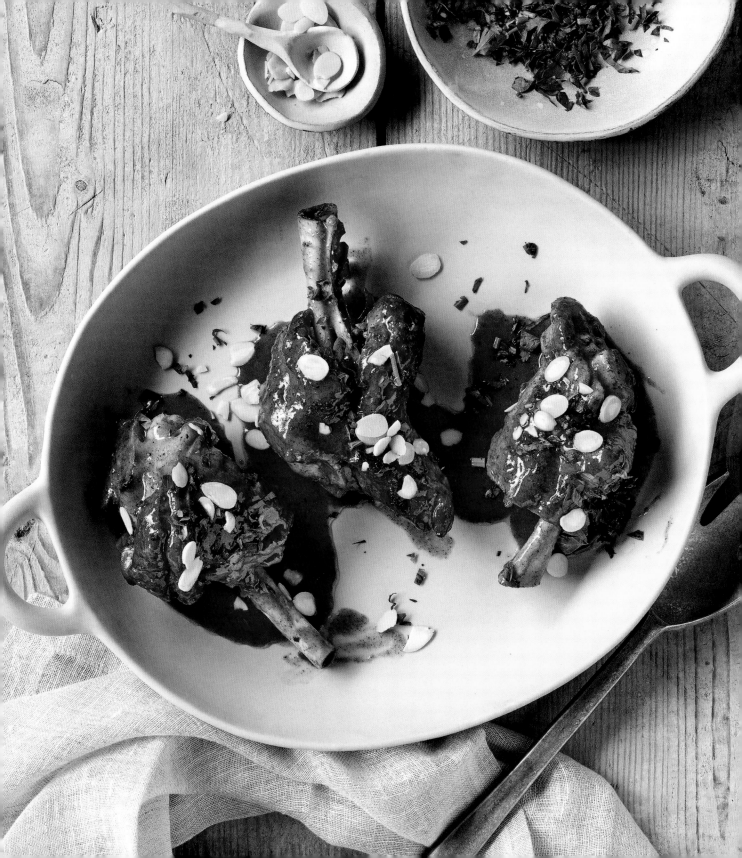

pan and bring to a simmer over medium heat. Cook until the sauce has reduced by about half, 15 to 20 minutes.

In a small bowl, whisk the arrowroot starch with 1 tablespoon cold water until the arrowroot has dissolved. Pour the arrowroot mixture into the sauce and stir until the sauce has thickened, about 2 minutes. Return the lamb shanks to the pot and stir to coat with the sauce. Cook until warmed through, about 3 minutes.

Arrange the lamb shanks on a serving platter. Spoon over the remaining sauce and garnish with the almonds and parsley.

SINIYEH BITAHEENA (SEASONED LAMB BAKED WITH TAHINI)

There's a small restaurant called Jerusalem that's just around the corner from where Catalina's parents live in midtown Toronto. (Actually, the restaurant has two locations, but that's beside the point.) They serve standard Middle Eastern fare, and things like *kofta kebab*, *shish tawook*, and Jerusalem mix grill dot the menu. Inconspicuously tucked among the other offerings is a dish called *siniyeh bitaheena*, described as "seasoned ground lamb and beef mixed with onions and parsley, oven baked with taheena sauce, garnished with pinenuts and almonds."

My experience of eating this for the first time many years ago has yet to escape me. It arrives at your table in a small, piping-hot, tin-pie-dish-looking vessel. As you work your spoon into the molten tahini, you reveal a bed of perfectly seasoned lamb. It's almost as though you're digging for buried treasure. Over the past year or so, I've been playing with re-creating a version of this dish at home with the hopes of sharing a similar experience with the reader.

In a large bowl, combine the lamb, onion, garlic, parsley, salt, coriander, Aleppo pepper, cumin, and black pepper. Mix with your hands until just combined. Cover and refrigerate for at least 6 hours or up to overnight.

Preheat the oven to 425°F.

Divide the mixture between two 8-inch pie dishes and flatten it into an even layer using your hands. Roast, uncovered, for 8 to 10 minutes, until the meat is cooked through. Pour the tahini over the top and return the pans to the oven. Roast for 3 minutes more.

Garnish with parsley leaves and the toasted almonds and serve immediately.

1½ pounds ground lamb (you can substitute ground beef, if you like)

1 large yellow onion, finely chopped

4 garlic cloves, finely chopped

¼ cup loosely packed fresh parsley leaves, finely chopped, plus more for garnish

2 teaspoons kosher salt

1½ teaspoons ground coriander

1 teaspoon Aleppo pepper or red pepper flakes

½ teaspoon ground cumin

½ teaspoon freshly ground black pepper

½ cup tahini

¼ cup unsalted slivered almonds, toasted, for garnish

Gluten-Free

Dairy-Free

Whole30

Keto-Friendly

Paleo

Grain-Free

Sugar-Free

Time: 30 minutes, plus 6 hours of marinating

PORK & LAMB

155

GREEK LAMB BURGERS

Time: 25 minutes, plus at least 30 minutes of marinating

2 pounds ground lamb

½ red onion, finely chopped (about ½ cup), plus about ½ cup more for serving

½ large green bell pepper, finely diced (about ½ cup)

½ cup loosely packed fresh parsley leaves, finely chopped

¼ cup pine nuts, toasted

2 garlic cloves, finely chopped

1 teaspoon dried mint

1 teaspoon dried oregano

2 tablespoons avocado oil, for drizzling

Kosher salt and freshly ground black pepper

4 heads iceberg lettuce (see headnote)

½ cup Bootleg Garlic Sauce (page 234), for serving

1 large hothouse or beefsteak tomato, thinly sliced, for serving

4 sugar-free dill pickles, thinly sliced into ribbons, for serving

½ cup kalamata olives, pitted and coarsely chopped

These aren't your average Greek burgers. In addition to the usual suspects (ground lamb, garlic, onion, dried oregano, and fresh parsley), I include dried mint, green bell pepper, and toasted pine nuts. The mint adds a delicious herbaceous flavor, the bell pepper lends a bit of sweetness and juiciness to the meat, and the pine nuts bring an unexpected crunch to the table.

Contrary to popular belief, you don't need any binders or fillers such as bread crumbs to keep your burgers from falling apart. As long as your meat has enough fat in it (I like a ground meat that is between 25 and 30 percent fat) and you push out as much air as possible from the patty, you shouldn't have any worries. I use what I call the "baseball and glove" technique to remedy the latter problem.

Start by forming a ball with the ground meat mixture. Then, pretend the ball of meat is a baseball and that you have a catcher's mitt on one hand. Hold the meatball using your free hand and proceed to "whip" it into the other hand (the one wearing the imaginary mitt), kind of like you would if you were tossing a baseball into a glove. This will help expel air trapped in the meat. After doing this a few times, form the ball into a patty. I hope that's a clear enough picture. After that, I use my thumb to make a small indentation in the center of each patty to prevent the burger from puffing up when cooking. The latter is an invaluable tip I learned in J. Kenji López-Alt's book *The Food Lab*.

When it comes to making the lettuce "buns," I prefer to use iceberg. It's crunchy and holds its shape, especially when cutting it the way I describe. You can expect to get 2 "buns" from a head of iceberg, so for four burgers, you'll need two heads of lettuce. You can, of course, also enjoy these burgers between your favorite bun, gluten-free or otherwise, or as a protein on top of a salad. Better yet, try pairing them with my Oven Fries (page 200) and Civilake Tizaki (page 236) to keep the Greek flavors flowing.

recipe continues

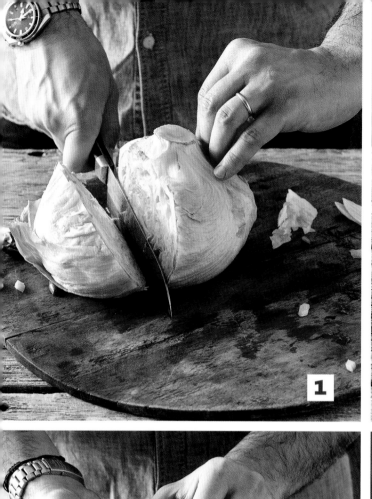

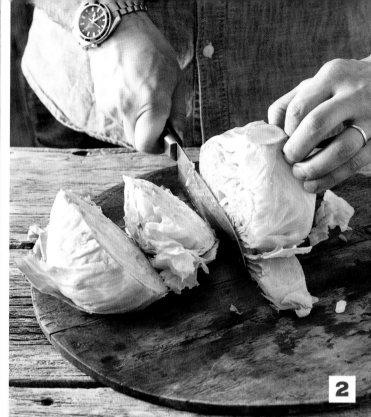

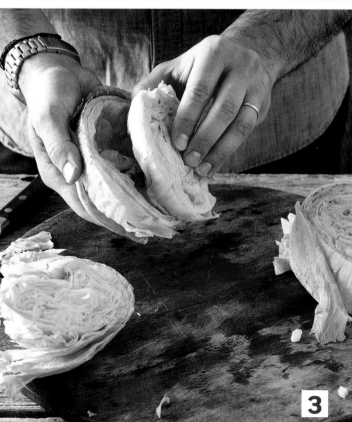

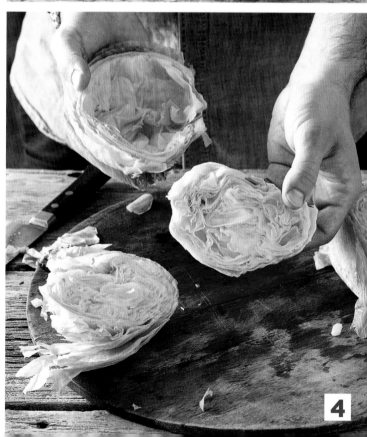

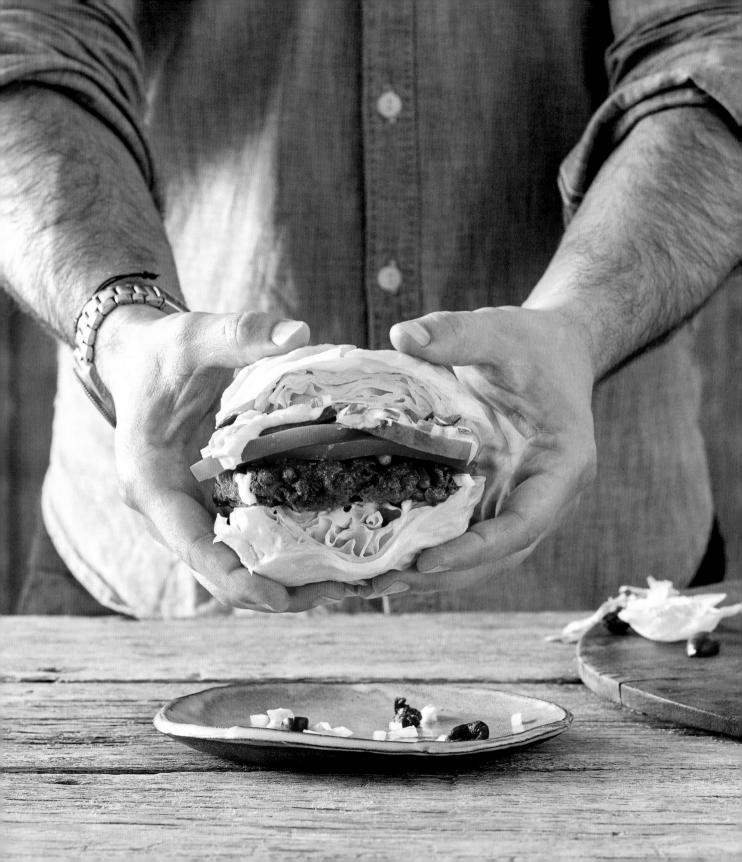

Line a rimmed baking sheet with parchment paper.

In a large bowl, combine the lamb, onion, bell pepper, parsley, pine nuts, garlic, mint, and oregano. Mix with your hands until just combined (overworking the meat can cause it to toughen).

Divide the mixture into 8 meatballs weighing approximately 4 ounces each. Form the balls into patties (see the "baseball and glove" technique outlined on the previous page) and use your thumb to make a small indentation in the center of each. Transfer the patties to the prepared baking sheet, cover with plastic wrap, and refrigerate for at least 30 minutes or up to overnight to allow the flavors to come together. (At this point, you can freeze the patties: if freezing, separate each patty with a sheet of parchment paper or waxed paper, stack them in a freezer-safe plastic bag, and freeze for up to 6 months.)

Heat a grill to medium-high or heat a grill pan over medium-high heat.

Drizzle both sides of each patty with 1 teaspoon of the avocado oil and liberally season with salt and pepper. Cook the burgers until grill marks form, flipping once, until cooked to your desired doneness, about 4 minutes per side.

For the lettuce "buns," place the head of lettuce stem-side up and use a knife to cut along either side of the core—you should be left with two outer pieces and a center disc. Reserve the center piece for another use, if you'd like. Using your hands, pull out the inner part of each cut piece so that you are left with a top and bottom bun.

Serve the burgers buffet-style with the lettuce buns, garlic sauce, tomato, pickles, and olives.

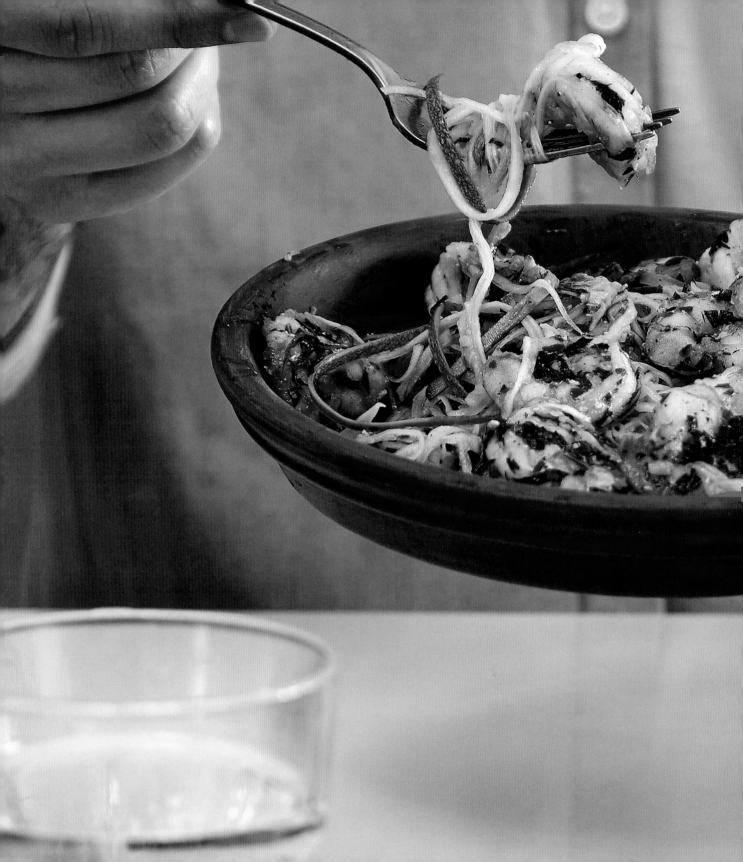

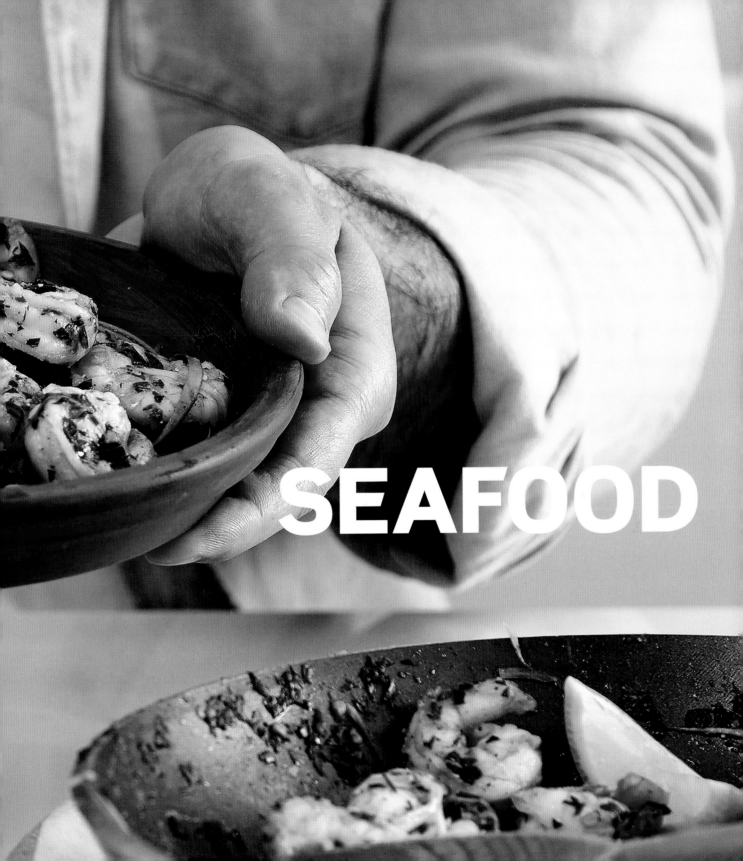

SEAFOOD

ADOBO SHRIMP
WITH CAULIFLOWER "GRITS" AND COLLARD GREENS

Gluten-Free
Dairy-Free
Whole30
Keto-Friendly
Paleo
Grain-Free
Sugar-Free

Time: 45 minutes

For the Cauliflower Grits:

1 head cauliflower, cut into florets

¼ cup full-fat coconut milk

2 tablespoons extra-virgin olive oil

½ teaspoon kosher salt, plus more as needed

For the Collard Greens:

1 tablespoon kosher salt, plus more as needed

1 pound collard greens (about 1 bunch), leaves stemmed and coarsely chopped

2 tablespoons avocado oil

2 garlic cloves, finely chopped

Freshly ground black pepper

For the Adobo Shrimp:

¾ pound raw jumbo shrimp (21/25 count), peeled and deveined

2 tablespoons Adobo Seasoning (page 254)

2 tablespoons avocado oil

This is a healthy spin on one of my all-time favorite comfort foods: shrimp and grits. Use any size shrimp you like—for me, the bigger, the better. If you're not a fan of collard greens, Garlicky Rapini (page 211) or Sautéed Tuscan Kale with Pine Nuts (page 196) are excellent substitutions. In fact, feel free to substitute just about any wilted green you like here.

MAKE THE CAULIFLOWER GRITS: In a large pot fitted with a steamer basket, bring 2 cups water to a boil over high heat. Add the cauliflower to the steamer basket, cover, and cook until the florets are tender, 10 to 12 minutes.

Carefully transfer the steamed cauliflower to a food processor, reserving the cooking liquid in the pot. To the food processor, add the coconut milk, olive oil, and salt and pulse until combined. Scrape down the sides of the food processor with a spatula and process until smooth and creamy but not runny. If the mixture is too thick for your taste, add 1 tablespoon of the reserved cooking liquid. Taste and adjust the seasoning as desired. Transfer the grits to a serving bowl and cover to keep warm until ready to serve.

MAKE THE COLLARD GREENS: Bring a large pot of water to a boil over high heat. Season with the salt, add the collards, and cook until softened, 10 to 12 minutes. Transfer the greens to a colander to drain completely.

recipe continues

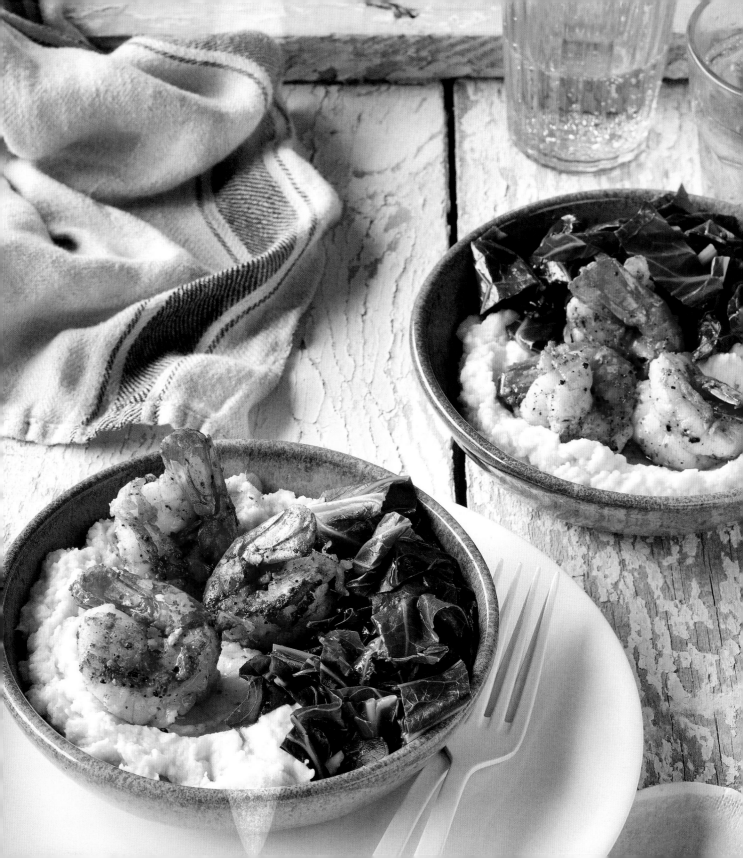

In a large stainless-steel or nonstick skillet, heat the avocado oil over medium-low heat. Add the garlic and cook, stirring, until fragrant, about 2 minutes. Add the drained collards and cook, stirring occasionally, until warmed through, 3 to 4 minutes. Taste and season with more salt and some pepper, if desired. Cover with a lid to keep warm and set aside until ready to serve.

MAKE THE ADOBO SHRIMP: In a medium bowl, combine the shrimp and adobo seasoning and toss to coat.

In a nonstick skillet, heat the avocado oil over medium-high heat. Add the shrimp and cook until pink and cooked through, about 3 minutes per side.

To serve, spoon the cauliflower grits into individual bowls. Top with the shrimp and collard greens and serve immediately.

MEDITERRANEAN CALAMARI

Don't get me wrong, there's nothing I love more than crispy fried calamari! But believe me when I tell you that calamari is also delicious when sautéed. I've been making calamari this way for years. It was first inspired by a Euro-trip my wife and I took back in 2010. We ate our way through Italy on the last leg of our journey, and I remember having a sautéed calamari dish somewhere along the Amalfi Coast, near Positano, I think. Long story short, the flavors have stuck with me and I've been trying to re-create it ever since.

This makes for an excellent appetizer since all the ingredients can be prepared ahead of time and it only takes around 10 minutes to cook. If, however, you'd like to make this a main course, you can simply double the ingredient quantities and serve it with some boiled potatoes alongside. Just be sure to use a large enough skillet so that you don't crowd the calamari and cause it to steam rather than sauté.

Pat the calamari dry with a paper towel. Using the tip of a very sharp knife, gently score one side of each calamari in a crosshatch pattern. Set aside.

Put the olive oil, shallot, and garlic in a large stainless-steel or non-stick skillet. Cook over medium-high heat, stirring, until the shallot is soft and translucent, 2 to 3 minutes. Add the calamari (including the tentacles, if using) and cook, tossing regularly, for about 2 minutes. Add the sun-dried tomatoes, capers, red pepper flakes, oregano, and a pinch each of salt and black pepper and cook until the calamari are slightly firm, 1 to 2 minutes. Add the vinegar and cook, stirring and scraping up any browned bits from the bottom

¾ pound calamari, with tentacles, if possible

3 tablespoons extra-virgin olive oil

1 shallot, thinly sliced

1 garlic clove, finely chopped

2 tablespoons sliced sun-dried tomatoes packed in oil, drained

1 tablespoon capers packed in brine, drained

Pinch of red pepper flakes

Pinch of dried oregano

Kosher salt and freshly ground black pepper

1 tablespoon balsamic vinegar

1 tablespoon fresh parsley leaves, for garnish

2 or 3 lemon wedges, for garnish

Gluten-Free
Dairy-Free
Whole30
Keto-Friendly
Paleo
Grain-Free
Sugar-Free

Time: 20 minutes

recipe continues

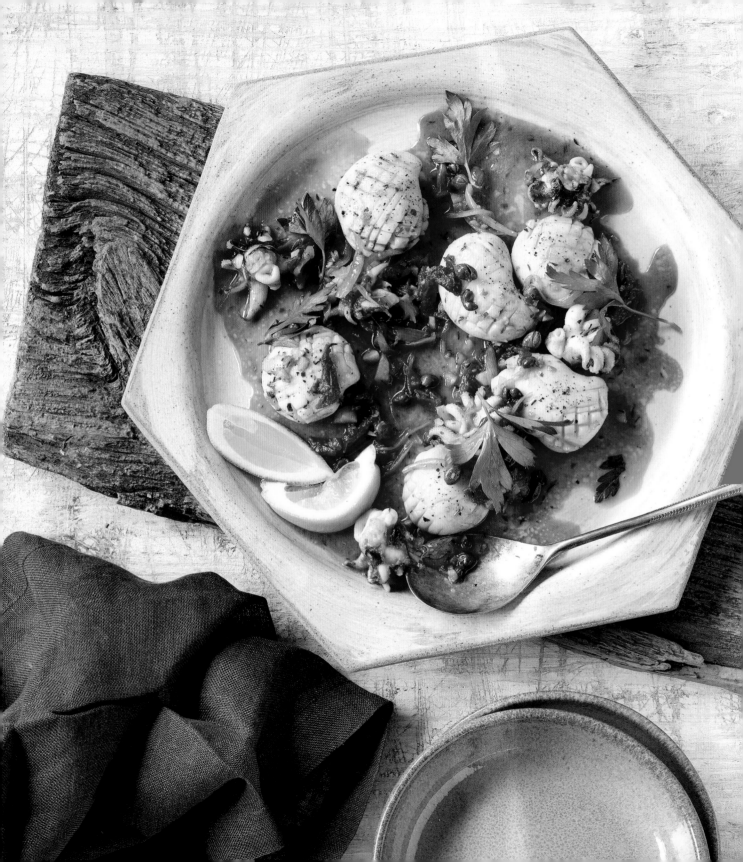

of the pan, until the liquid has slightly reduced, about 2 minutes. Taste and season with more salt and black pepper, if desired.

Lay the calamari in a serving bowl, scored-side up. Spoon the pan sauce and any tentacles over the top and garnish with the parsley. Serve with the lemon wedges for spritzing. Enjoy immediately.

Note: Gradually heating the shallot and garlic over medium heat will not only infuse the oil with flavor, but will also help prevent them from burning.

SHRIMP SCAMPI

Gluten-Free
Dairy-Free
Whole30
Keto-Friendly
Paleo
Grain-Free
Sugar-Free

Time: 15 minutes

2 tablespoons finely chopped garlic (about 3 large cloves)

1 tablespoon ghee

1 tablespoon extra-virgin olive oil

¾ pound raw jumbo shrimp (21/25 count), peeled, tails on, and deveined

1 teaspoon red pepper flakes (optional)

⅓ cup chicken stock

1 tablespoon fresh lemon juice

Kosher salt and freshly ground black pepper

¼ cup loosely packed fresh parsley leaves, finely chopped

This is an effortless scampi that is delicious on its own, incredible over some Perfect Zucchini Noodles (page 188), and killer when spooned over a grilled steak for some surf-and-turf action.

In a large stainless-steel or nonstick skillet, combine the garlic, ghee, and olive oil. Cook over medium-high heat, stirring, until the garlic is fragrant, about 2 minutes. Pat the shrimp very dry with a paper towel. Add them to the pan and cook, stirring, until slightly pink, about 2 minutes per side. Add the red pepper flakes (if using) and cook, stirring, for 1 minute.

Add the stock and lemon juice and cook until the liquid has reduced by about a quarter, about 2 minutes. Taste the sauce and season with salt and black pepper. Remove the pan from the heat and stir in the parsley. Serve immediately.

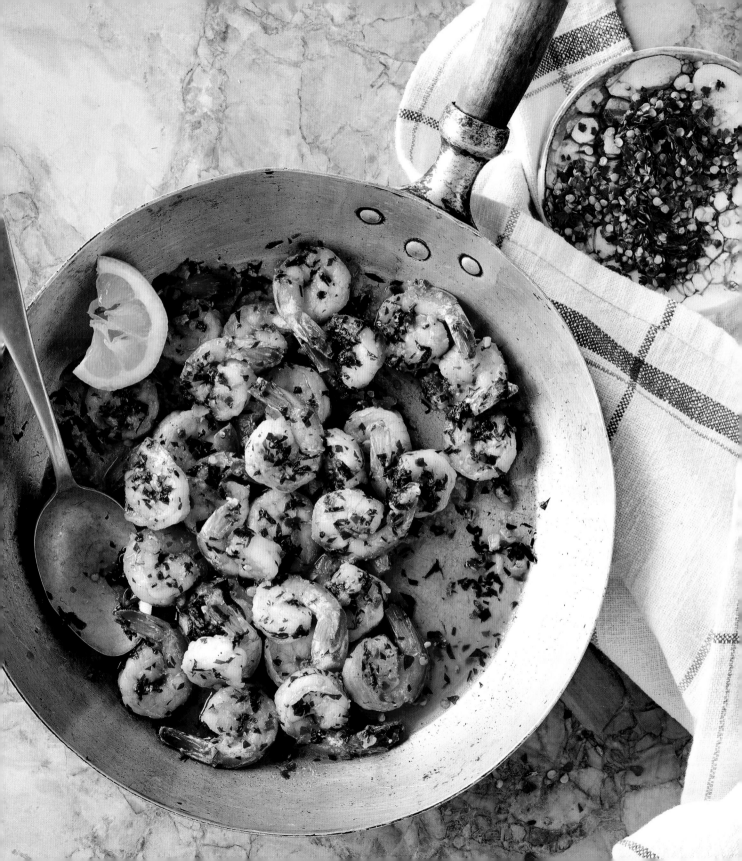

SAUTÉED SHRIMP
WITH WARM PICKLED PEPPERS

Gluten-Free

Dairy-Free

Whole30

Keto-Friendly

Paleo

Grain-Free

Time: 25 minutes

¾ pound raw jumbo shrimp (21/25 count), peeled, tails kept on, and deveined

1 tablespoon Adobo Seasoning (page 254)

1 tablespoon avocado oil

1 small carrot, cut into thin matchsticks

½ red bell pepper, cut into thin matchsticks

½ green bell pepper, cut into thin matchsticks

½ yellow onion, thinly sliced

½ Scotch bonnet chile, seeded and finely chopped

½ teaspoon whole allspice berries

¼ cup distilled white vinegar (or white wine vinegar, sherry vinegar, or rice vinegar)

1 to 3 teaspoons agave syrup or honey

This is inspired by an outrageously delicious dish I had in Negril, Jamaica. We were there celebrating my brother's bachelor party and had booked a day of fishing. The only thing I caught was a case of seasickness, but one of our friends hooked some beautiful yellowfin tuna. We brought it back to the resort and asked one of the chefs to help us prepare it. He seasoned the fish with a yellowish powder, which I later came to learn was Vegeta, and sautéed some peppers and onions in a spicy vinegar sauce, which is referred to as *escovitch* in Jamaica (or *escabeche* in Spain and the Philippines).

Here I replace the fish with shrimp, but you could substitute snapper, haddock, halibut, or cod. The peppers are spicy, light, and bursting with an unexpected twang from the vinegar. I've also replaced the additive-heavy Vegeta seasoning blend with my Adobo Seasoning. You'll definitely need the agave or honey to balance the acidity, so perhaps it's best to keep this dish for your Food Freedom. Try serving it with some Twice-Fried Plantains (page 218), Sweet Plantains (Maduros) (page 210), Cauliflower Rice (page 205), or steamed rice.

Pat the shrimp dry with a paper towel and lightly season them on both sides with the adobo seasoning.

In a medium nonstick skillet, heat the avocado oil over medium-high heat. Add the shrimp and cook until pink and firm, 2 minutes per side. Transfer the shrimp to a plate and set aside.

In the same skillet, combine the carrot, bell peppers, onion, Scotch bonnet, and allspice berries. Cook, stirring, until the vegetables have softened slightly, 2 to 3 minutes. Add the vinegar, honey (use 1 teaspoon for a less sweet version), and ¼ cup water. Cook until the liquid has reduced by half, about 5 minutes. Taste and season with salt as desired.

Spoon the pickled peppers and sauce onto a serving platter and top with the sautéed shrimp. Garnish with the avocado wedges and cilantro leaves and serve.

Kosher salt

1 avocado, cut into wedges, for serving

2 tablespoons fresh whole cilantro leaves, for serving

PAN-FRIED SALMON
WITH MUSTARD-DILL CREAM SAUCE

Gluten-Free

Dairy-Free

Whole30

Keto-Friendly

Paleo

Grain-Free

Sugar-Free

Time: 20 minutes

2 (8-ounce) skinless salmon fillets, about 1 inch thick

1 teaspoon sweet Spanish paprika (see Notes)

Kosher salt and freshly ground black pepper

1 tablespoon extra-virgin olive oil

2 garlic cloves, finely chopped

1 cup full-fat coconut milk

2 tablespoons fresh lemon juice, plus more if needed

1 tablespoon Dijon mustard

1 tablespoon capers packed in brine, drained

¼ cup loosely packed fresh dill, finely chopped

In this recipe, salmon fillets get pan-fried and browned to perfection before being smothered in a quick-and-easy dairy-free cream sauce. It takes only 15 minutes to cook, so it's an absolutely perfect back-pocket weeknight lean protein option and can be easily adjusted to serve a crowd. Try serving it with a side of leafy greens and boiled potatoes.

Pat the salmon fillets dry with paper towels. Lightly season both sides with the paprika and salt and pepper.

In a large nonstick skillet, heat the olive oil over medium-high heat. Gently lay the fish in the hot oil and cook until the fish is medium-rare and the center of each fillet reads 110°F on an instant-read thermometer, about 2½ minutes per side. Transfer the salmon to a plate or baking sheet, tent with aluminum foil, and set aside.

Discard all but 1½ tablespoons of the fat from the skillet. Return the skillet to medium-high heat, add the garlic, and cook, stirring, for 30 seconds. Stir in the coconut milk, lemon juice, mustard, and capers. Cook, stirring regularly, for 4 minutes. Remove the skillet from the heat and stir in the dill. Taste the sauce and adjust the seasoning with more pepper and lemon juice, if desired. Return the salmon to the sauce to gently warm it, then serve.

Notes: For a bit of heat, try substituting hot paprika or add a touch of cayenne pepper when seasoning the salmon.

Since the capers have a bold, briny flavor, it is important to just lightly season each salmon fillet with salt.

You can also use skin-on fillets here. If so, I recommend cooking them skin-side down for 3½ minutes to develop a crispy crust and then 1½ minutes on the flesh side to finish. Also, be sure to return the salmon to the sauce flesh-side down so the skin does not get soggy.

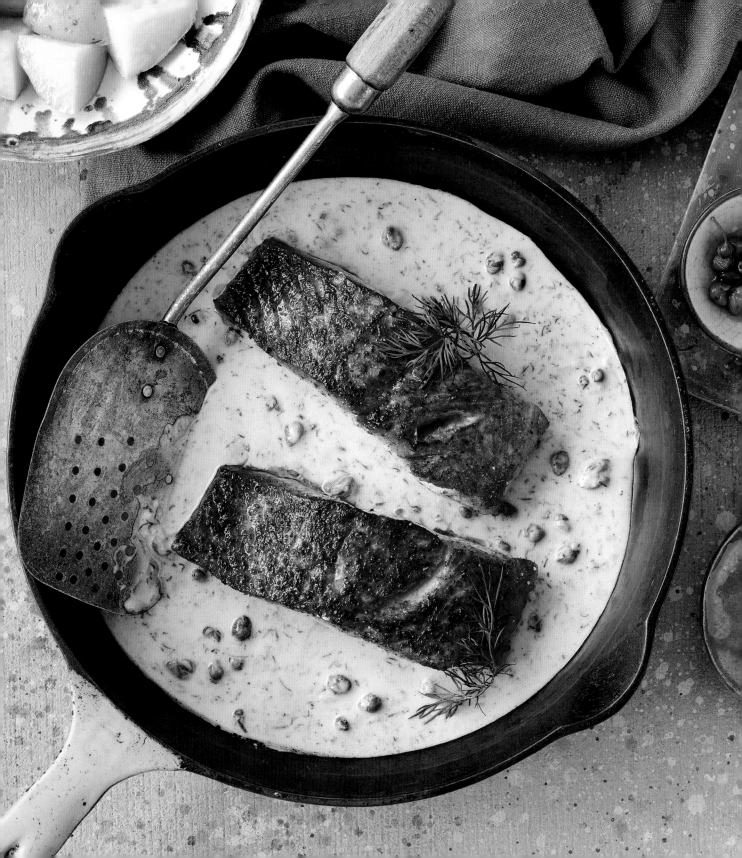

ASIAN ROAST SALMON
WITH CASHEWS

Gluten-Free

Dairy-Free

Paleo

Grain-Free

Time: 35 minutes, plus at least 1 hour of marinating

¼ cup coconut aminos

2 garlic cloves, finely chopped

1 tablespoon Dijon mustard

1 tablespoon toasted sesame oil

1 tablespoon pure maple syrup (omit for Whole30)

1½ teaspoons grated fresh ginger

1 (2-pound) side of salmon, scaled and boned

¼ cup raw unsalted cashews, coarsely chopped

2 scallions, white and light green parts only, thinly sliced

Topping roasted salmon with nuts may sound unusual, but trust me when I tell you it works! If you can't find a whole side of salmon, then feel free to use individual fillets—just keep in mind that they'll cook more quickly. Try serving the roasted fish over some Cauliflower Rice (page 205) or in lettuce cups.

In a medium bowl, combine the coconut aminos, garlic, mustard, sesame oil, maple syrup, and ginger and whisk until smooth. Place the salmon in a zip-top plastic bag, add the marinade, and massage to coat. Seal the bag and refrigerate for 1 to 4 hours.

Meanwhile, in a dry skillet, toast the cashews over medium heat until golden brown, about 5 minutes. Set aside.

Position racks near the top and bottom of the oven and preheat to 375°F.

Remove the salmon from the marinade, letting any excess drip off. Discard the remaining marinade. Place the salmon skin-side down in a roasting pan or rimmed baking sheet. Transfer the salmon to the bottom rack of the oven and cook until the thickest part registers 115°F on an instant-read thermometer for medium-rare, about 20 minutes.

Set the oven to broil.

Transfer the salmon to the top rack of the oven. Cook until the top of the salmon is golden brown and it reads 125°F internally, about 5 minutes more.

Garnish with the toasted cashews and the scallions. Serve immediately.

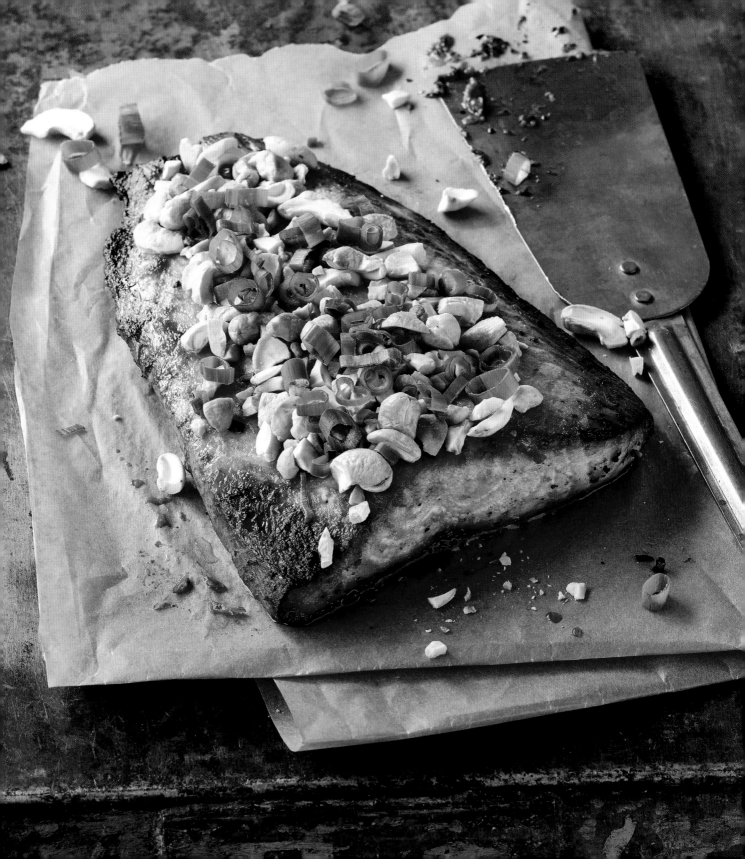

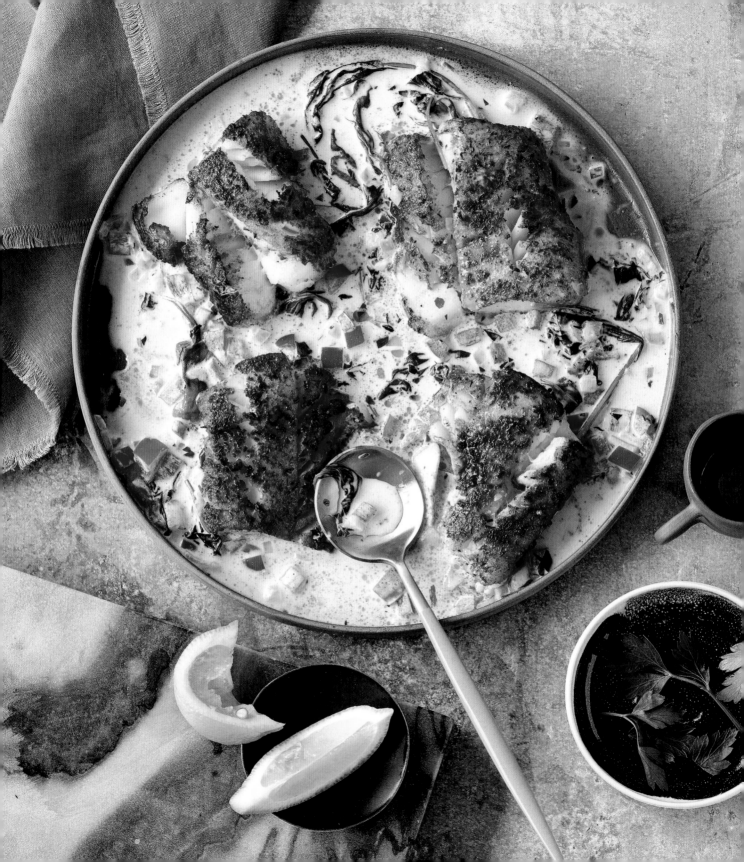

CAJUN COD
WITH RED PEPPER AND SPINACH CREAM SAUCE

Raw cod, not the salted kind, is an incredibly versatile fish. It is fairly mellow in flavor, lends itself to a variety of recipes, and can often be found wild-caught, usually from Iceland. It's also usually more affordable than other white-fleshed fish, like haddock, halibut, or hake. Just keep in mind that it can be a bit delicate, so handle it with care when cooking, and be sure to let a crust develop on one side before trying to flip it. If cod or other types of white-fleshed fish are unavailable, you can substitute salmon. To round out the meal, try serving the fish with some boiled or mashed potatoes.

Pat the cod fillets dry with a paper towel. Lightly season both sides of each fillet with the Cajun seasoning.

In a large nonstick skillet, heat the olive oil over medium-high heat. Gently lay the fish in the hot oil and cook until the fish is medium-rare and the center of each fillet reads 110°F on an instant-read thermometer, about 2½ minutes per side. Transfer the cod to a plate or baking sheet, tent with aluminum foil, and set aside.

Discard all but 1½ tablespoons of the oil from the skillet. Return the skillet to medium-high heat, add the bell pepper and shallot, and cook, stirring, until they begin to soften, about 2 minutes. Add the garlic and cook, stirring, for 1 minute. Stir in the coconut milk and lemon juice and cook, stirring regularly, until the sauce has reduced by one-quarter, about 4 minutes. Add the spinach and parsley and cook, stirring occasionally, until the spinach has just wilted, 1 to 2 minutes. Taste the sauce and adjust the seasoning with salt and more lemon juice, as desired. Return the cod fillets to the sauce to gently warm through, then serve.

2 (8-ounce) or 4 (4-ounce) cod fillets, about 1 inch thick

1 tablespoon Ragin' Cajun Spice Rub (page 259)

1 tablespoon extra-virgin olive oil

½ red bell pepper, diced

1 shallot, diced

2 garlic cloves, finely chopped

1 cup full-fat coconut milk

2 tablespoons fresh lemon juice, plus more if needed

2 cups packed baby spinach

¼ cup loosely packed fresh parsley leaves, finely chopped

Kosher salt

Gluten-Free
Dairy-Free
Whole30
Keto-Friendly
Paleo
Grain-Free
Sugar-Free

Time: 25 minutes

MIRACLE FISH AND CHIPS
WITH TARTAR SAUCE

Gluten-Free

Dairy-Free

Grain-Free

Sugar-Free

Time: 35 minutes

½ cup avocado oil, plus more as needed

8 (4-ounce) boneless, skinless fresh or thawed white-fleshed fish fillets (see discussion at right)

½ cup Miracle Batter (page 247)

Kosher salt

Oven Fries (page 200), for serving

1 cup Whole30 Tartar Sauce (page 245), for serving

1 lemon, cut into wedges, for serving

I think it was on Fridays that my high school cafeteria would serve fish and chips. Greasy, deep-fried, overseasoned white fish would be served with a side of fries and a tablespoon of tartar sauce. It was gross, but to be honest, I just couldn't get enough of it. I would spend the rest of the afternoon staring blankly at my desk, my brain fog so thick that I had a hard time staying awake, let alone getting any work done. Maybe that's why I failed calculus twice and did even worse the second time? (Or maybe I'm just bad at math. . . .)

These fish and chips are a cleaned-up version of that cafeteria dish, one of my childhood favorite eats. The Miracle Batter is grain-free, gluten-free, and dairy-free, but gets unbelievably crispy while staying superlight and airy. If you didn't know any better, you'd think the Oven Fries were, well, fried! Technically speaking, the battered-and-fried fish and fries are made with Whole30-compliant ingredients. However, I would file this under "SWYPO" (see page xxii) because both the fish and the chips are Paleo versions of common junk foods. They might even fall under "Foods with No Brakes" for you. I have to admit that I personally have a hard time resisting second or even third helpings, so this dish is something best enjoyed during your Food Freedom.

As far as sauce pairings go, I can't imagine having fish and chips without some creamy and delicious tartar sauce. Just like the fish and chips, the Tartar Sauce is a cleaned-up version and makes use of my 30-Mississippi Mayonnaise. It's Whole30-compliant, so feel free to serve it with other dishes like my Chicken Schnitzel (page 40). Just be sure to read the ingredients on the dill pickles to ensure they're sugar- and alcohol-free.

You can use a variety of white-fleshed fish here. Halibut, haddock, Pacific rockfish, and cod are all great options. If you want

recipe continues

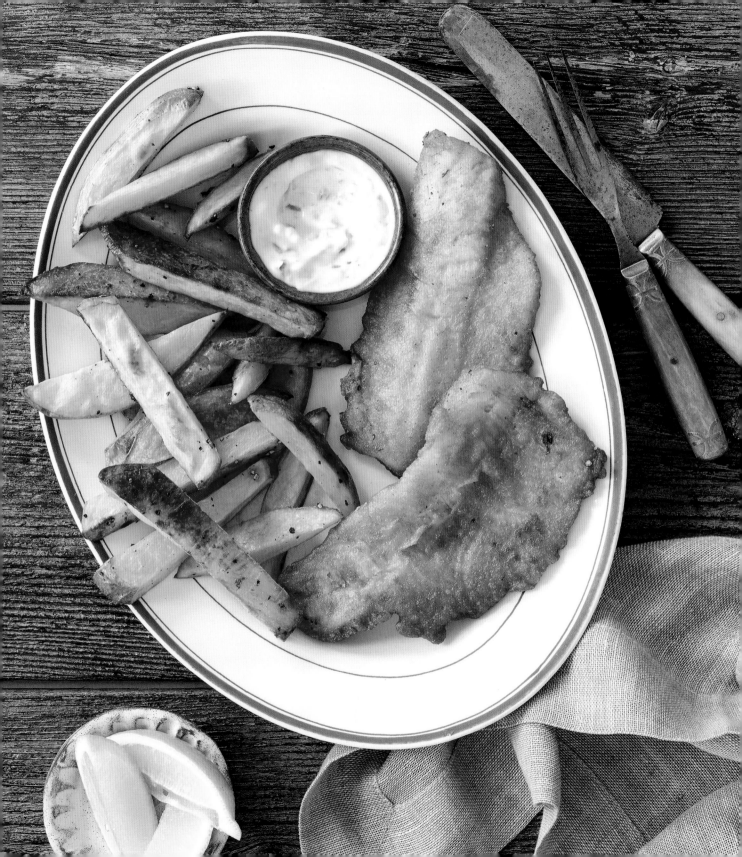

Notes: It's best to use fresh fish here. If using frozen, thaw it completely first, or it will cause the temperature of the oil to drop significantly, resulting in a greasy and soggy finished product. Also be sure to pat the fish dry so the batter sticks a bit better.

Unless you're making a big batch, three servings or more, fry the fish in batches in a medium pan, between 8 and 10 inches, rather than a large cast-iron one. A smaller pan will let you use less oil and will force the oil up along the sides of the fish. Since you'll be shallow frying, the fish will inevitably make contact with the bottom of the pan. A cast-iron pan retains heat better and distributes it more evenly than a nonstick pan, which are important considerations when frying, but a nonstick material will safeguard against the fish potentially sticking to the bottom of the pan. I also find that cast iron absorbs some of the oil.

to try something new, I highly recommend monkfish, if you can find it fresh. What monkfish lacks in looks (google it to get a visual), it makes up for in texture and taste. It's meaty and flavorful and doesn't fall apart on you like cod. It's also reasonably priced and often sustainably sourced. Ask your fishmonger to remove any membrane on the fillets, if they haven't already.

Preheat the oven to 225°F.

In a large nonstick skillet, heat ¼ cup of the avocado oil over medium heat to 350°F. Line a baking sheet with paper towels and place it near your frying station.

Working in batches, dredge the fish in the Miracle Batter and gently shake off any excess. Carefully lay the fish in the hot oil and cook until the fish is golden brown, crispy, and cooked through, 4 to 5 minutes per side. Transfer the fish to the lined baking sheet and immediately season with a pinch of salt. Place the baking sheet in the warm oven while you dredge and fry the remaining fillets, adding more oil to the pan between batches as needed.

Serve the fish with the fries, tartar sauce, and lemon wedges.

ROCK SHRIMP

Catalina and I used to go to this all-you-can-eat sushi restaurant called Sushi D in Toronto's Little Italy. For a while, it was the best bang-for-your-buck spot, especially since we were a couple of broke students trying to make it through grad school. The fish was fresh, the dishes tasted great, and the service was quick. Over time, however, the service slowed down, the food wasn't the same, and the prices went up.

In addition to all the sushi and maki, the thing to order was the rock shrimp. I'm not entirely sure if they used actual rock shrimp, or even how they prepared them, for that matter, but if I had to guess, the shrimp were battered, fried, and quickly tossed in a garlicky aioli. In a word, they were addictive. We'd order six portions at a time, knowing full well the restaurant gave only three or four shrimp per serving.

I've always wanted to re-create this recipe in a Paleo- and Whole30-friendly way, and thanks to my Miracle Batter (page 247)—which gets super crispy when fried, but tastes light and airy—I can relive those memories, except without the food coma that always followed.

In a large bowl, whisk together the mayonnaise and garlic. Cover and set aside.

In a large nonstick skillet, heat the avocado oil over medium heat to 350°F. Line a baking sheet or plate with paper towels and place it near your frying station.

Working in batches, dredge the shrimp in the Miracle Batter and gently shake off any excess. Carefully lay the shrimp in the hot oil and cook until golden brown, crispy, and cooked through, 2 to 3 minutes per side. Transfer the fried shrimp to the lined baking sheet and repeat to dredge and fry the remaining shrimp.

While the shrimp are still hot, add them to the bowl of garlicky mayo and toss to coat. Garnish with the chives and serve immediately.

¼ cup 30-Mississippi Mayonnaise (page 230)

1 garlic clove, finely chopped

¼ cup avocado oil

¾ pound raw jumbo shrimp (21/25 count), peeled and deveined

¼ cup Miracle Batter (page 247)

1 tablespoon finely sliced fresh chives, for garnish

Gluten-Free
Dairy-Free
Paleo
Grain-Free
Sugar-Free

Time: 30 minutes

CALAMARI PUTTANESCA

Gluten-Free
Dairy-Free
Whole30
Keto-Friendly
Paleo
Grain-Free
Sugar-Free

Time: 25 minutes

¾ pound calamari, sliced into rings and with tentacles (optional) separated

3 tablespoons extra-virgin olive oil

4 anchovy fillets packed in olive oil, chopped into a paste

1 shallot, thinly sliced

2 garlic cloves, finely chopped

¼ teaspoon red pepper flakes

1 (13.5-ounce) can crushed tomatoes

10 black olives, such as kalamata, pitted and coarsely chopped

2 tablespoons thinly sliced sun-dried tomatoes packed in olive oil, drained

1 tablespoon capers packed in brine, drained

Freshly ground black pepper

1 recipe Perfect Zucchini Noodles (page 188)

2 tablespoons finely chopped fresh parsley leaves

Pasta puttanesca is a Neapolitan red sauce made from tomatoes, anchovies, capers, and olives. *Puttanesca* literally translates to "in the style of a prostitute." The origins of the name remain shrouded in mystery, but the name itself has stuck, along with a very clear understanding of what should and shouldn't go into the dish.

Puttanesca is usually served with spaghetti, but I've also seen it paired with other types of noodles and even tube-shaped pasta, such as rigatoni. I like to serve it over my Perfect Zucchini Noodles (page 188), but you should feel free to experiment with whatever "pasta" you like. Whether it's a gluten-free rice flour noodle or a bowl of spaghetti squash, remember that you're the boss, applesauce.

On that note, I like to play with a recipe and make it my own. After all, I'm the one who has to eat it! In this case, I particularly like the addition of shallots and sun-dried tomatoes, which you don't usually find in the sauce for puttanesca. As for the calamari, it happens to lend itself quite nicely to the other ingredients in the sauce and is a nice break from the usual lean sources of protein. I think each ingredient brings something to the table in terms of flavor and texture. Purists will undoubtedly disagree, but that's perfectly fine.

Dry the calamari thoroughly with paper towels and set aside.

In a large stainless-steel or nonstick skillet, combine the olive oil, anchovies, shallot, and garlic. Cook over medium-high heat, stirring, until the shallot is soft and translucent, 2 to 3 minutes. Add the red pepper flakes and cook, stirring, for 1 minute more.

Add the crushed tomatoes, olives, sun-dried tomatoes, and capers. Season with black pepper and cook until the sauce has reduced

recipe continues

by one-quarter, 4 to 5 minutes. Add the calamari and cook, stirring regularly, until the calamari is opaque and firm, 3 to 4 minutes. Taste and adjust the seasoning as desired. Remove the pan from the heat, add the zucchini noodles and parsley, and toss to coat. Serve immediately.

Note: If you can find them, try using crushed cherry tomatoes. They will likely be sweeter than your average can of crushed tomatoes, and that sweetness will help balance the salt, acidity, and spice of the other ingredients in the sauce.

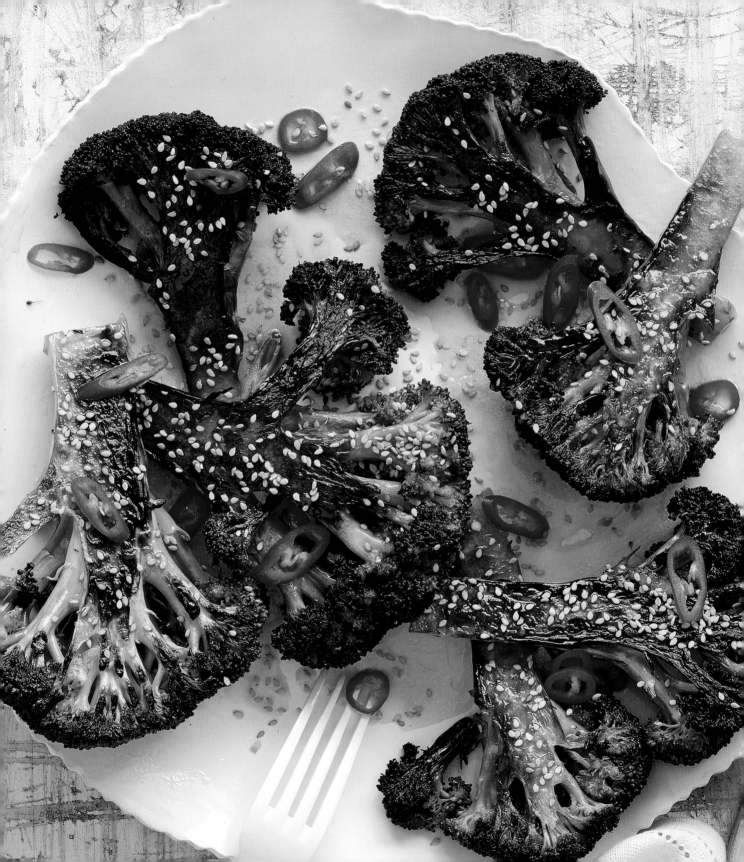

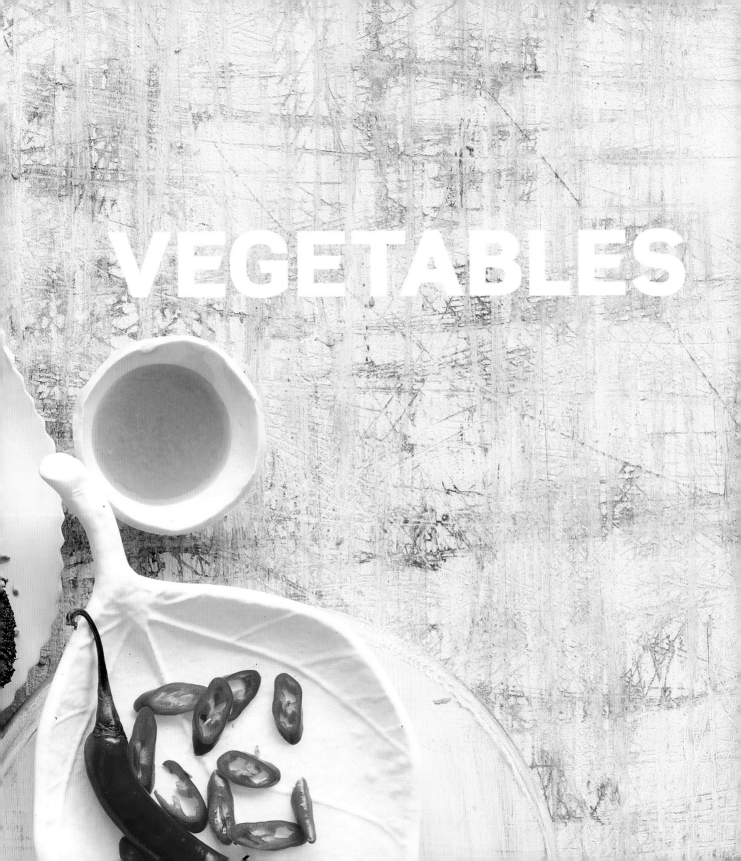

VEGETABLES

MAPLE-SESAME ROASTED CARROTS

Gluten-Free
Dairy-Free
Whole30
Paleo
Grain-Free

Time: 40 minutes

2 tablespoons avocado oil

3 garlic cloves, finely chopped

¼ cup coconut aminos

1 tablespoon pure maple syrup (omit for Whole30)

1 tablespoon toasted sesame oil

6 large carrots (about 2 pounds), cut into 2-inch pieces on an angle

2 scallions, white and light green parts only, thinly sliced, for garnish

2 teaspoons mixed black and white sesame seeds, for garnish

Flaky sea salt, for garnish

A delicious, Asian-inspired twist on roasted carrots that's perfect as a side for a Sunday roast. A little bit of maple syrup goes a long way and helps the carrots caramelize as they roast, but it's optional and can be omitted if you're doing a round of Whole30; the coconut aminos are fairly sweet themselves. You really want a bit of color on the carrots. They taste delicious with that slight bit of char! Just be careful not to completely burn them to a crisp.

Preheat the oven to 400°F. Line a baking sheet with parchment paper.

In a large stainless-steel or nonstick sauté pan, combine the avocado oil and garlic. Cook over medium-high heat, stirring, until the garlic starts to sizzle, 2 to 3 minutes. Stir in the coconut aminos, maple syrup, and sesame oil and cook for 1 minute. Add the carrots, toss to coat, and cook until the sauce has reduced by one-quarter, 2 to 3 minutes.

Using a slotted spoon, transfer the carrots to the prepared baking sheet and arrange them in a single layer. Drizzle half the pan sauce over the carrots, reserving the other half in the pan.

Roast the carrots for 20 to 22 minutes, until lightly charred and soft.

While the carrots roast, return the sauté pan to medium heat and cook until the sauce has reduced by half, about 4 minutes.

Transfer the roasted carrots to a serving platter and drizzle them with the sauce. Garnish with the scallions, sesame seeds, and a pinch of flaky salt and serve.

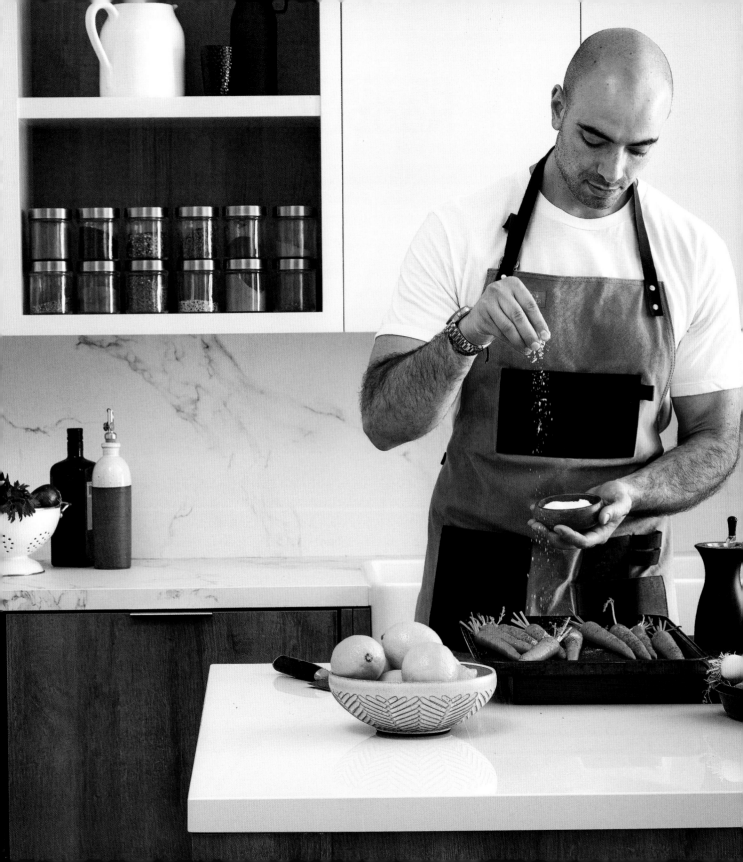

PERFECT ZUCCHINI NOODLES

Gluten-Free

Dairy-Free

Whole30

Keto-Friendly

Paleo

Grain-Free

Sugar-Free

Time: 35 minutes

4 zucchini

1 teaspoon
kosher salt

Tired of soggy zucchini noodles? You know, the ones that leave a pool of sour green liquid at the bottom of the bowl? Well, there's a way to avoid that and make perfect zucchini noodles every single time!

SPIRALIZE THE ZUCCHINI: I know, this is an obvious step, but have you ever considered the integrity of your noodle? You want long, luxurious strands of "zpaghetti" that dance between your mouth and the plate and don't fall apart. As much as I loathe the thought of wasting valuable storage space (and money) on kitchen gadgets that perform singular tasks—what Alton Brown calls "unitaskers"—I have to admit that a good spiralizer makes a world of difference here.

Look for one that comes with different blade attachments, a base with a suction cup to hold it in place on your counter, and a high clearance so that you can spiralize directly onto a plate or into a bowl.

SALT YOUR ZUCCHINI NOODLES: This, ladies and gentlemen, is the secret to perfect zoodles! Zucchini is loaded with water, which it will release once it comes into contact with salt or heat. To avoid a pool of slightly bitter green liquid at the bottom of your zpaghetti Bolognese, season your zucchini noodles with a pinch of salt (kosher or other) and massage all the strands to coat. Then place the zucchini noodles in a colander set over a bowl and wait. In just a few minutes, liquid will start to drain into the bowl. After about 30 minutes, most of the liquid will have drained. If you need to speed things up or you're working with a large batch of zucchini noodles, you can help the process along by gently squeezing the noodles (keep in mind that this will probably crush them a bit) and patting them dry with paper towels.

recipe continues

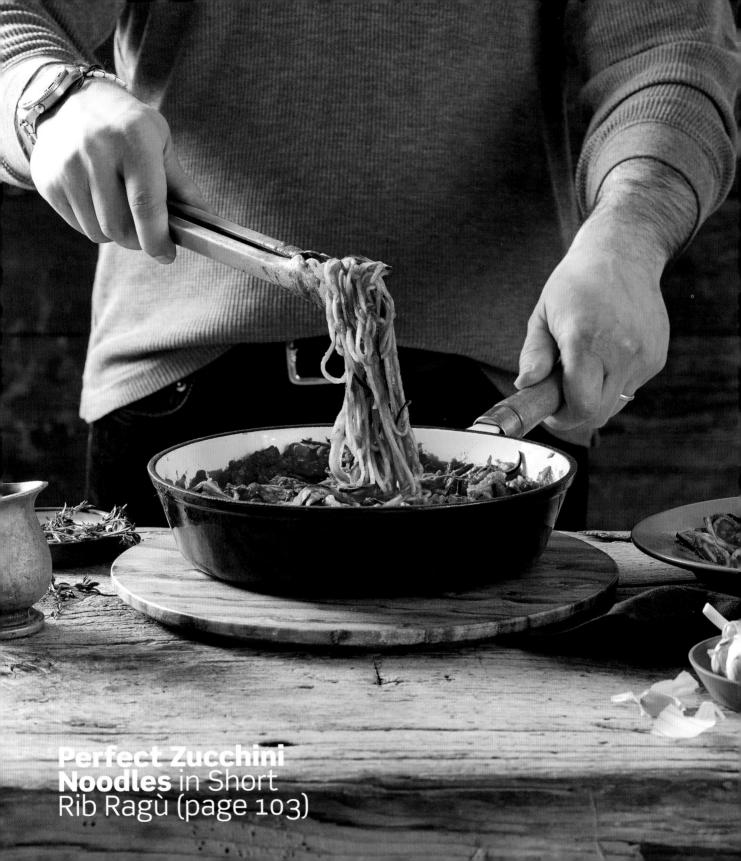

Perfect Zucchini Noodles in Short Rib Ragù (page 103)

DO NOT COOK ZUCCHINI NOODLES: Zucchini is perfectly edible raw, so cooking it is not entirely necessary. Instead, try warming them up by tossing them in whatever sauce you'll be serving them with. For example, if you're making Short Rib Ragù (page 103), add the drained zucchini noodles to a pan with the sauce, remove from the heat, and toss to coat. The residual heat from the sauce and the pan will be enough to warm the zucchini noodles without compromising their al dente texture.

Follow these steps, and you'll end up with a perfect, toothsome bite of zucchini noodles that will surprise even the biggest zoodle skeptics.

Trim the ends of the zucchini and pass them through a spiralizer to create noodles. Transfer the zucchini noodles to a colander set over a bowl, sprinkle with the salt, and massage the noodles to coat. Let the zucchini noodles sit until drained of excess moisture, about 30 minutes, or up to 1 hour. Drain the zucchini noodles and serve as desired.

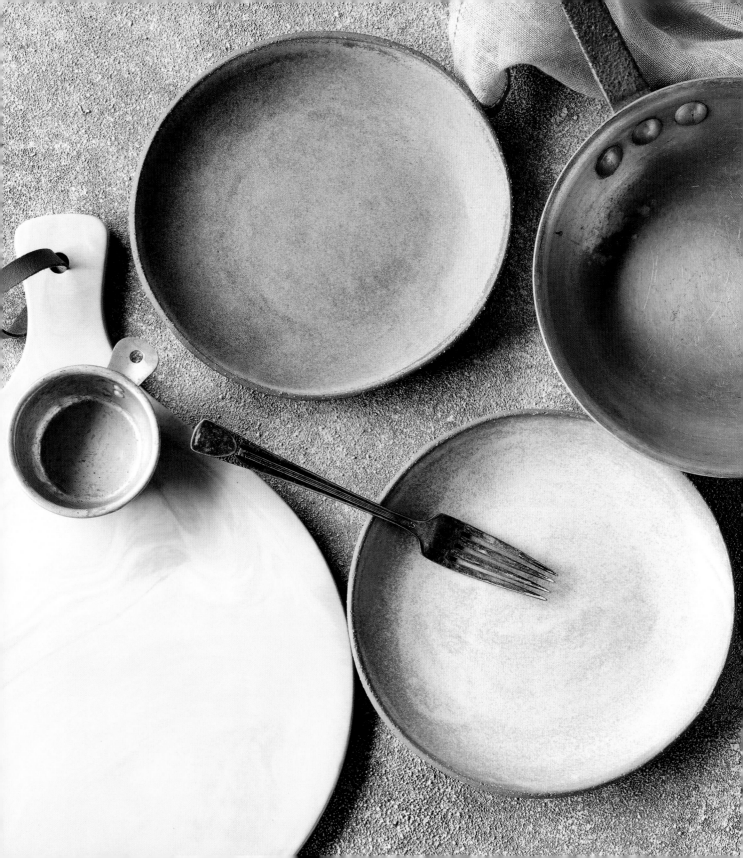

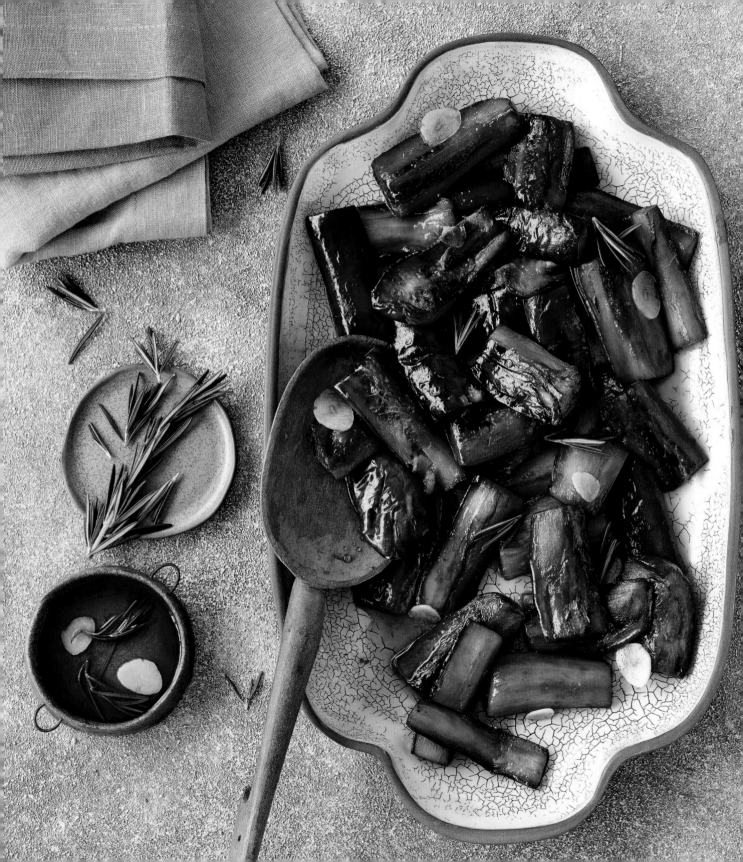

EGGPLANT AGRODOLCE

Agrodolce is a lovely Italian sweet-and-sour sauce that is as delicious to say as it is to eat. It's commonly used as a condiment to glaze grilled pork chops, chicken, or fish, but works just as well with vegetables. It's typically made with equal parts vinegar and sugar. Here I keep things Paleo by substituting maple syrup, a natural sweetener. You could just as easily use honey, but I'm Canadian, and maple syrup flows through my veins.

In a small saucepan, combine the vinegar, maple syrup, garlic, and rosemary. Cook gently over medium-low heat, stirring occasionally, until the agrodolce is reduced and syrupy, 10 to 12 minutes.

Meanwhile, in a large nonstick skillet, heat the olive oil over medium-high heat. Add the eggplant and cook, stirring frequently, until browned and softened, 12 to 15 minutes. Add the agrodolce to the pan with the eggplant and toss to coat. Cook for 2 to 3 minutes more so the sauce sticks to the eggplant.

Transfer to a serving platter and serve immediately.

¼ cup white balsamic vinegar (or rice vinegar or white wine vinegar)

¼ cup pure maple syrup

3 garlic cloves, thinly sliced

1 tablespoon loosely packed fresh rosemary, finely chopped

3 tablespoons extra-virgin olive oil

3 Japanese eggplant, halved lengthwise and cut into 2-inch pieces

Gluten-Free
Dairy-Free
Paleo
Grain-Free

Time: 25 minutes

VEGETABLES

HERB-AND-GARLIC-STUFFED PORTOBELLO MUSHROOMS

Gluten-Free

Dairy-Free

Whole30, if modified

Keto-Friendly

Paleo

Grain-Free

Sugar-Free

Time: 30 minutes

4 large portobello mushroom caps

¼ cup grass-fed butter or ghee, at room temperature

¼ cup finely chopped fresh parsley leaves, plus more for garnish

1½ teaspoons finely chopped garlic

Kosher salt and freshly ground black pepper

A fast, no-fuss, delicious mushroom side dish that presents beautifully on the table. Make a quick compound butter with some garlic and fresh parsley, and slather it all over big, juicy portobello mushrooms. Roast them hot and fast to get rid of their excess moisture, and brown the butter or ghee.

Preheat the oven to 425°F. Line a rimmed baking sheet with parchment paper.

Wipe the mushrooms clean with a damp paper towel and place them gill-side up on the prepared baking sheet.

In a medium bowl, stir together the butter, parsley, and garlic until well combined. Evenly spread the butter over the gill side of each mushroom and season each with a pinch each of salt and pepper. Bake until the mushrooms are deeply browned and sizzling, 22 to 25 minutes. Garnish with parsley and serve immediately.

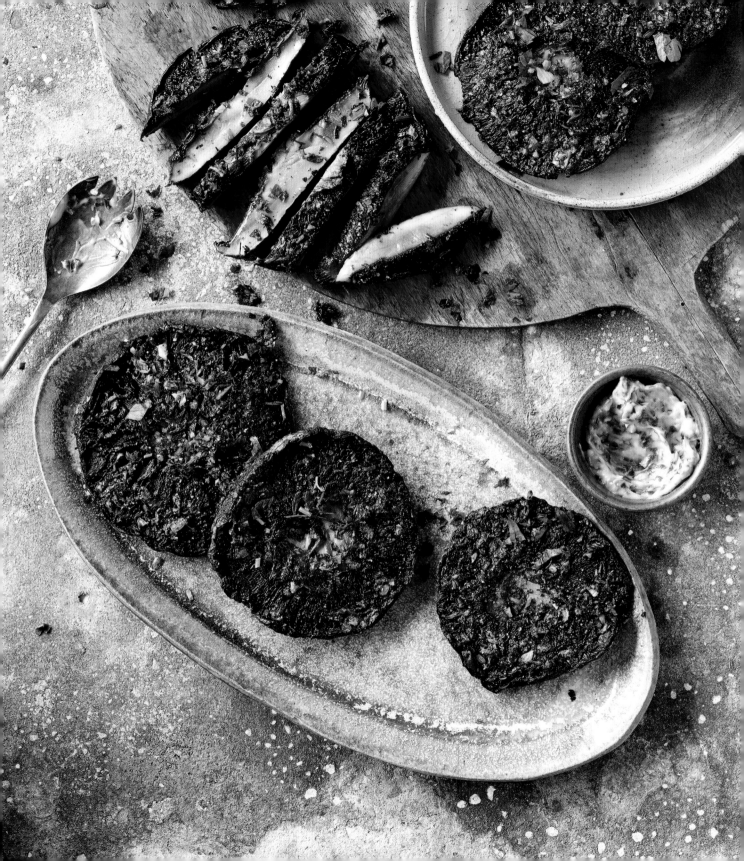

SAUTÉED TUSCAN KALE
WITH PINE NUTS

Gluten-Free

Dairy-Free

Whole30

Keto-Friendly

Paleo

Grain-Free

Sugar-Free

Time: 25 minutes

1 pound Tuscan kale (also called cavolo nero, lacinato kale, or dinosaur kale; about 1 bunch)

Kosher salt

¼ cup pine nuts

3 tablespoons extra-virgin olive oil, plus more for finishing

2 garlic cloves, thinly sliced

1 teaspoon red pepper flakes

½ lemon, cut into wedges, for serving

I love this sautéed Tuscan kale when it has a bit of bite to it, but if you'd like it softer, you have two options. The first is to cook it for longer—steam the kale for 8 to 10 minutes instead of the 3 minutes called for. The other option is to blanch the kale in a pot of salted boiling water before sautéing. Doing this will also make the kale less bitter, which you may prefer. Personally, I like the mild bitterness, especially when I'm enjoying these greens with a fatty grilled rib eye steak!

If you'd like to try blanching first, start with this step and continue as normal. You can also just skip the blanching step and go straight to sautéing.

Trim the lower parts of the kale stems and use your hands to strip the leaves from the stems. Finely chop the stems and set aside. Stack the leaves on top of one another, cut them crosswise into 1-inch ribbons, and set aside.

Fill a large bowl with ice and water and set it nearby.

Bring a large pot of water to a boil over high heat. Season the water with 2 tablespoons salt, add the kale leaves, and cook until tender and bright green, about 3 minutes. Transfer the kale to the ice water and let stand for 3 minutes to stop the cooking and set the vivid green color. Drain the kale very well before cooking.

In a large sauté pan, toast the pine nuts over medium heat until lightly browned and fragrant, 3 to 4 minutes. Transfer the nuts to a bowl or plate and set aside.

recipe continues

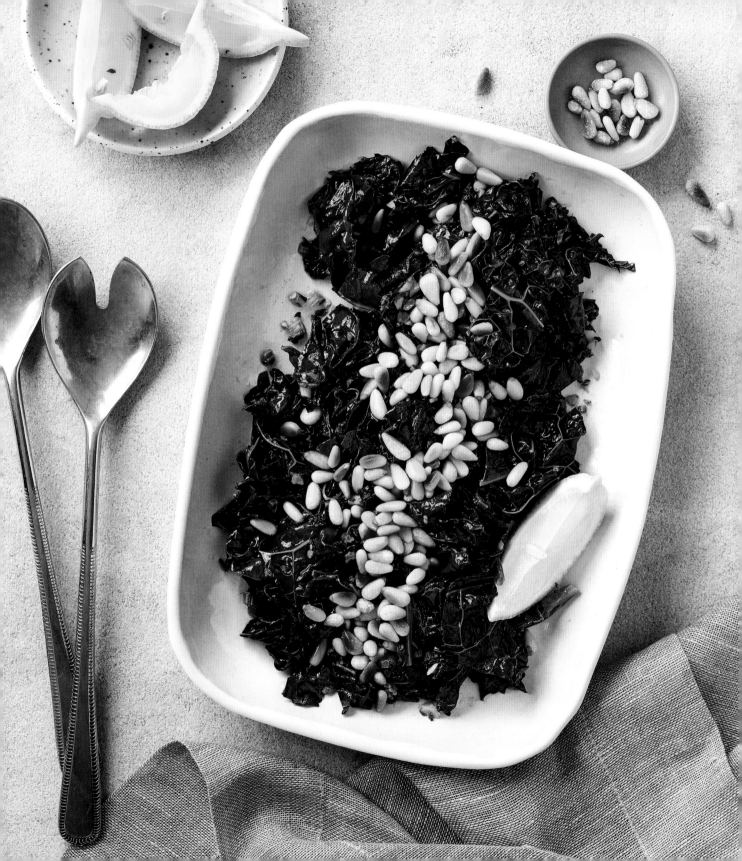

In the same pan, heat the olive oil over medium heat. Add the chopped kale stems and the garlic and season with a pinch of salt. Cook, stirring, until the kale stems soften, about 3 minutes. Add the red pepper flakes and cook for 1 minute. Add the kale leaves and season with another small pinch of salt. Toss the kale to coat in the oil. Add 2 tablespoons water and quickly cover the pan to trap the steam. Cook until wilted and tender, 3 minutes, stirring once about halfway through. Taste and adjust the seasoning.

Transfer the cooked kale to a serving platter, garnish with the toasted pine nuts, drizzle with a bit more olive oil, and serve with the lemon wedges alongside for squeezing over the top.

GARLICKY MASHED SWEET POTATOES

These mashed sweet potatoes have been a staple side dish in my house since I started my health journey. They're incredibly easy to prepare, can be adjusted to feed a crowd, and are almost impossible to mess up. Keep in mind that the time it takes for the sweet potato to cook depends on how big or small you cut them. I like to chop them up into 1-inch pieces to help speed things along. Don't worry about making the pieces perfectly uniform because everything gets mashed in the end anyway.

Bring a large saucepan of water to a boil over high heat. Season the water with 1 tablespoon salt and add the sweet potatoes. Boil until the potatoes are fork-tender, about 15 minutes, then drain them and return them to the pot.

Add the olive oil, garlic, and ghee (if using) to the pot with the sweet potatoes. Season with a pinch each of salt and pepper and mash the potatoes with a fork or potato masher until smooth.

Transfer the mashed sweet potatoes to a serving bowl, drizzle with a bit more olive oil, and season with a pinch of flaky salt. Serve immediately.

Kosher salt and freshly ground black pepper

4 sweet potatoes, peeled and cut into 1-inch cubes

3 tablespoons extra-virgin olive oil, plus more for finishing

2 garlic cloves, finely chopped

1 tablespoon ghee (optional)

Flaky sea salt, for finishing

Gluten-Free

Dairy-Free

Whole30

Paleo

Grain-Free

Sugar-Free

Time: 40 minutes

VEGETABLES

OVEN FRIES

Gluten-Free
Dairy-Free
Whole30
Grain-Free
Sugar-Free

Time: 45 minutes

2 pounds yellow or white potatoes

2 tablespoons avocado oil

¾ teaspoon kosher salt

¼ teaspoon freshly ground black pepper

I resisted regular potatoes for about two years in the beginning of my health journey, relying almost exclusively on low-glycemic sweet potatoes instead. I loved potatoes a little too much and found myself mindlessly binging on them whenever given the chance. This, in turn, led to a carb-induced crash that threw off my eating habits and energy levels for the rest of the day. So I decided it would be best to steer clear of them unless they were part of a treat meal.

It wasn't until my second round of Whole30 that I decided to reintroduce potatoes in a more thoughtful and consistent manner. At first, I limited them to a small amount at lunchtime and paid closer attention to how much of them I ate, how they made me feel while I was eating, and how I felt afterward. I also assessed whether I could do without them. For example, could I muster the willpower to leave a couple of potatoes behind to enjoy with dinner, or did I have to eat them all at once? Much to my surprise, I found that I didn't need to eat as many to enjoy them, and as a result, they didn't cause me to feel lethargic or bloated afterward.

Since then, potatoes of all kinds have become a staple starch in my diet, and these oven fries are one of the ways I love to enjoy them! They're every bit as crispy and delicious as their deep-fried cousins but won't leave you falling asleep on the couch in the middle of the day.

Preheat the oven to 425°F. Line a baking sheet with parchment paper.

Rinse and scrub the potatoes to remove any dirt. After patting them dry, cut them into ¼-inch-thick matchsticks and arrange them on the prepared baking sheet. Drizzle the avocado oil over the potatoes and season with about half the salt and all the pepper. Toss to coat, then spread the fries into a single layer over the baking sheet.

Roast on the bottom rack of the oven until the fries are golden brown and fork-tender, 30 to 35 minutes—no need to flip them halfway. Season with the remaining salt and serve immediately.

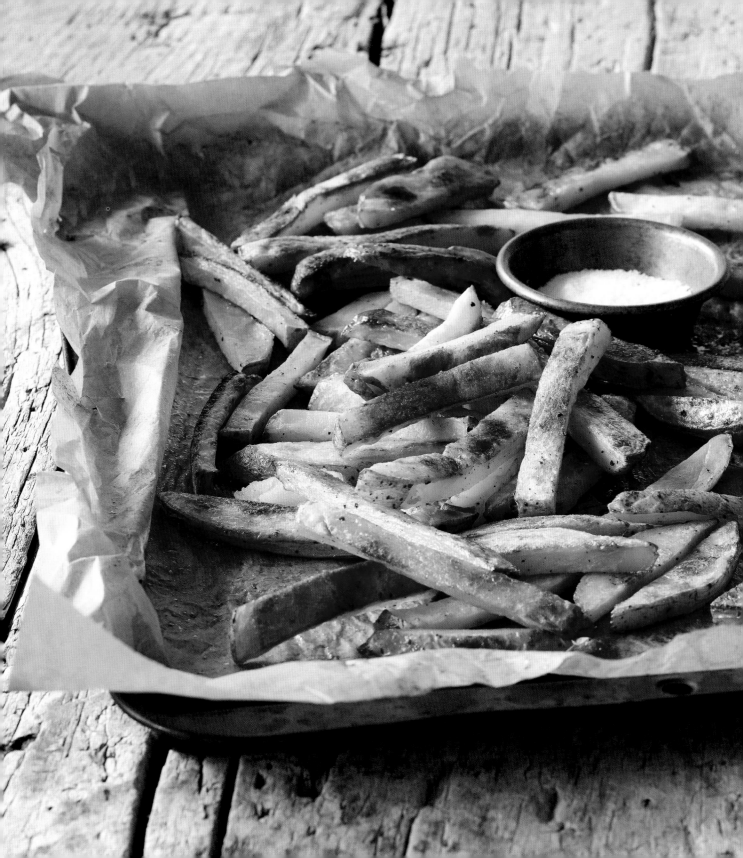

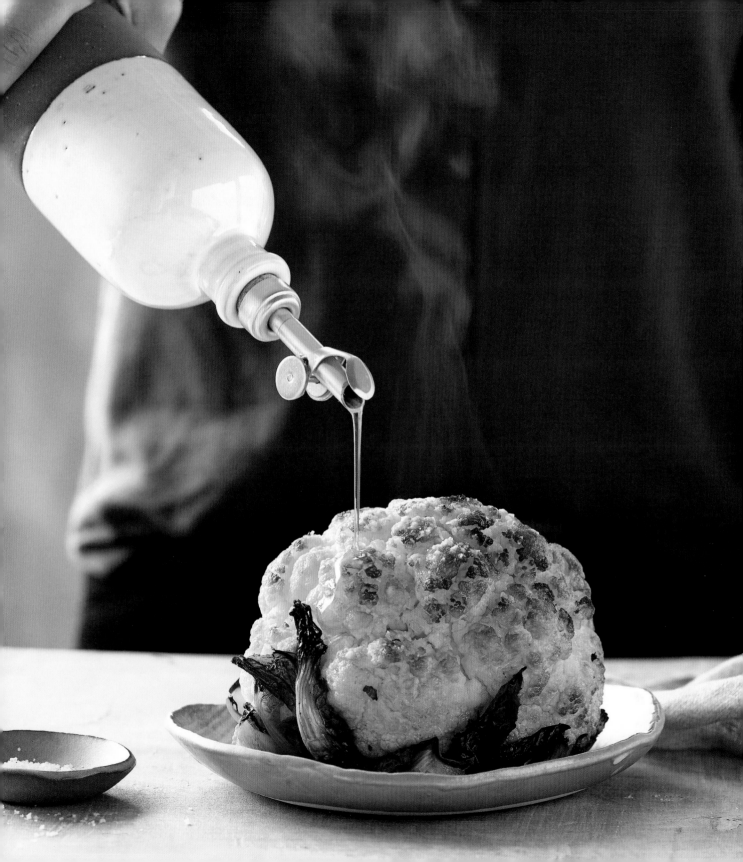

ROAST CAULIFLOWER

I had heard tales and seen pictures of Eyal Shani's empire of falafel shops, but I didn't realize he had an outpost in Vienna, so it was completely by accident that Catalina and I stumbled across Miznon while traveling in Vienna back in 2017. It was a very pleasant surprise when I walked past a restaurant window full of heads of cauliflower on that intensely hot summer day.

In many ways, Eyal Shani is part of the reason cauliflower is having its day in the sun. It was only after he started roasting and selling them whole that other chefs followed suit. Before long, restaurants were pushing for vegetable-forward menus and cauliflower became a staple item. Rightfully so, too. Cauliflower is versatile, beautiful, and delicious.

I tried again and again to reverse-engineer Miznon's famous whole-roasted cauliflower once we got home from the trip. I tried dry roasting, roasting with a water bath, steaming and then roasting, roasting at different temperatures, so on and so forth. After about a dozen tries, I felt as though I had finally cracked the Miznon cauliflower code. Of course, by that time, Eyal Shani had already publicly shared the recipe online with a variety of food magazines!

Much to my surprise, I was pretty close, and it turns out the key is to keep things very simple. I also found that it helps if you spread the florets apart a bit after parboiling the head of cauliflower. Not only does this allow some of the oil to slide down to the core of the cauliflower, it also lets hot air circulate through the vegetable for a more evenly cooked finished product. The only thing that sets this recipe apart is the fact that I rub it with a bit of ghee before roasting for added flavor and a bit more color.

Preheat the oven to 425°F. Line a baking sheet with parchment paper.

Trim the stem of the cauliflower so the cauliflower will stand upright on the board. If the cauliflower has leaves still attached, do not trim them off.

1 head cauliflower, preferably with leaves still attached

2 tablespoons plus 1 teaspoon kosher salt

2 tablespoons ghee, at room temperature

2 tablespoons extra-virgin olive oil

Flaky sea salt, for garnish

Gluten-Free

Dairy-Free

Whole30

Keto-Friendly

Paleo

Grain-Free

Sugar-Free

Time: 1 hour

recipe continues

Bring a large pot of water to a boil over high heat. Add 2 tablespoons of the salt and submerge the cauliflower in the water, stem-side up. Boil until the florets have slightly softened but are still intact, 10 to 12 minutes. Place the cauliflower stem-side down on a wire rack to drain and let air-dry for 5 minutes.

Stand the cauliflower on the prepared baking sheet and, using your hands, spread apart the florets to create some crevices. Rub the florets with the ghee and season with the remaining 1 teaspoon salt. Roast until the florets are golden brown and fork-tender, 40 to 45 minutes.

Drizzle the roasted cauliflower with the olive oil and finish with a sprinkle of flaky salt. Serve immediately.

CAULIFLOWER RICE

The easiest way to rice cauliflower is to pass it through the grater attachment on a food processor. If you don't have a food processor, use a box grater. If you don't have one of those, finely chop the cauliflower by hand. Whichever way you do it, you want to break down the cauliflower into pieces about the size of grains of rice. And no matter which method you choose, I strongly encourage you to drain the cauliflower of excess moisture by squeezing it in a clean kitchen towel or nut milk bag. Like zucchini, cauliflower holds a lot of water, and that liquid will be released once the vegetable is heated.

Feel free to serve this cauliflower rice as is, maybe alongside my Spicy Green Bean and Cashew Nut Chicken (page 79) or Picadillo (page 96). It can be customized any number of ways, too. Try adding flavor in the form of lime zest, chopped jalapeño, sautéed vegetables, coconut aminos, kimchi, etc. The world is your oyster! (I bet you thought I was going to say, "You're the boss, applesauce"!)

Grate the cauliflower using a food processor fitted with a grating blade or on the large holes of a box grater (alternatively, finely chop the cauliflower by hand into pieces roughly the size of grains of rice).

Transfer the riced cauliflower to a clean kitchen towel and bring the corners of the towel together. Wrap the cauliflower tightly and securely in the towel and twist to squeeze out as much moisture as possible. (Alternatively, you can use a nut milk bag for this step.)

In a large skillet, heat the avocado oil over medium heat. Add the cauliflower and cook, tossing regularly, until it starts to turn golden brown, about 6 minutes. Season with salt and serve.

1 head cauliflower, cut into 2-inch florets

2 tablespoons avocado oil

Kosher salt

Gluten-Free

Dairy-Free

Whole30

Keto-Friendly

Paleo

Grain-Free

Sugar-Free

Time: 15 minutes

ROAST CAULIFLOWER FLORETS WITH KALE AND WALNUT PESTO

Gluten-Free

Dairy-Free

Whole30

Keto-Friendly

Paleo

Grain-Free

Sugar-Free

Time: 35 minutes

1 head cauliflower, cut into 2-inch florets

2 tablespoons avocado oil

½ teaspoon kosher salt

¼ teaspoon freshly ground black pepper

¼ cup Kale and Walnut Pesto (page 238)

Roasted cauliflower florets are just one of the many things you can toss in my Kale and Walnut Pesto. It makes a delicious and easy-to-prepare side dish for any night of the week. Living your Food Freedom? Try this with a bit of freshly grated Parmigiano Reggiano, pecorino, or Grana Padano cheese on top.

Preheat the oven to 450°F. Line a baking sheet with parchment paper.

Spread the cauliflower florets over the prepared baking sheet, drizzle with the avocado oil, and season with the salt and pepper. Toss to coat. Arrange the florets in an even layer and roast until golden brown and slightly softened, 25 to 30 minutes.

Transfer the warm cauliflower to a medium bowl and toss with the pesto. Serve immediately.

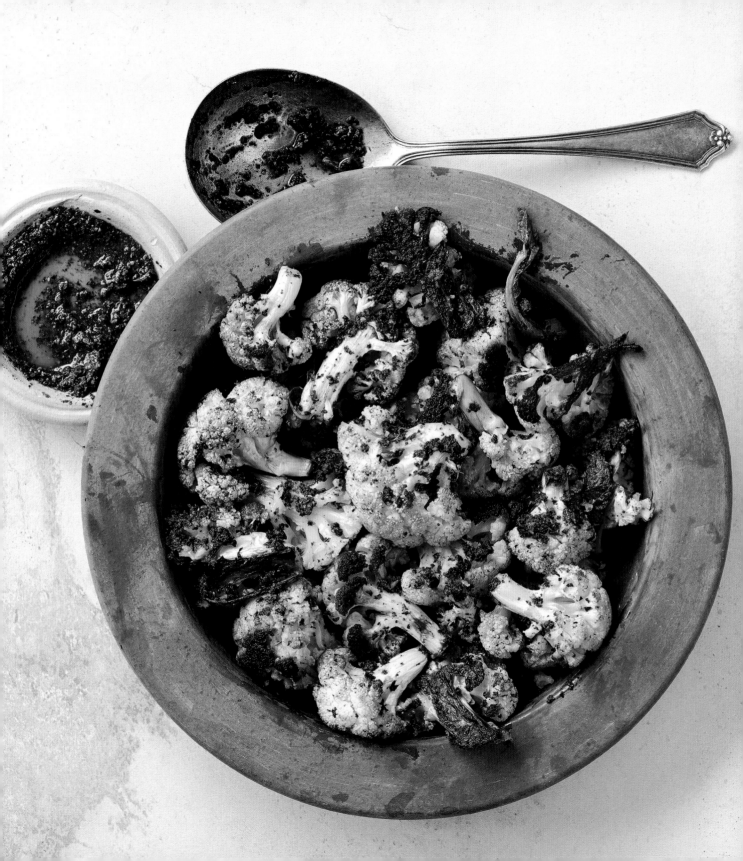

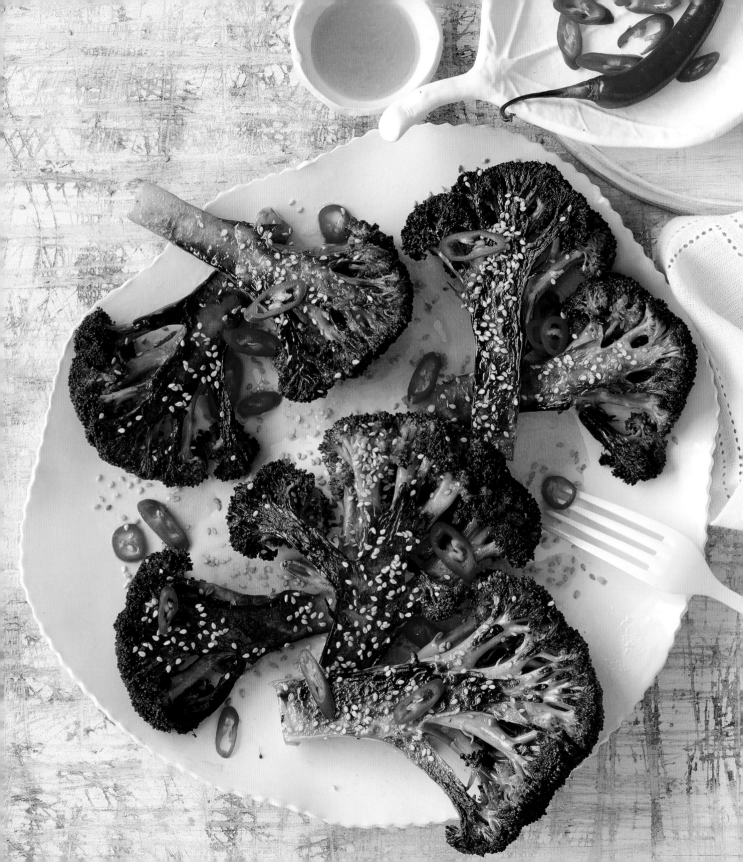

PAN-ROASTED BROCCOLI "STEAKS"
WITH GARLIC-SESAME VINAIGRETTE

This technique for pan-roasting broccoli "steaks" is adapted from an *America's Test Kitchen* recipe for Brussels sprouts. Here, I substitute broccoli crowns, which develop a beautifully caramelized crust as they simultaneously steam and tenderize.

The Asian-inspired vinaigrette has a touch of honey in it, making it off-limits for Whole30. Normally, I would simply suggest leaving it out if you're doing a round of Whole30, but you really need it here to balance the acidity of the vinegar and the bitterness of the broccoli. If you'd like to enjoy this during a round of Whole30, try it plain or pair it with another one of my Whole30-compliant sauces, such as Cha Cha Chimichurri (page 235), The Dracula Killer (Toum) (page 242), Uncle Ronny's Romesco (page 243), Tahini Sauce (page 240), or Zhug (page 246). I promise, the charred vegetable is delicious even on its own.

In a mason jar, combine the olive oil, vinegar, garlic, sesame oil, and honey. Seal the jar tightly and shake vigorously until emulsified. Set aside until ready to serve. (The vinaigrette can be stored in the refrigerator for up to 2 weeks.)

Pour the avocado oil into a large stainless-steel sauté pan and lay the broccoli in the oil in a single layer, cut-side down. Work in batches, if needed. Cover the pan with a lid, place it over medium-high heat, and cook until the bottoms of the broccoli start to turn golden, about 5 minutes. Remove the lid and cook until the bottoms are charred, 4 to 5 minutes more.

Arrange the broccoli steaks on a serving platter, drizzle them with the vinaigrette, and garnish with the sliced chile and sesame seeds. Serve immediately.

3 tablespoons extra-virgin olive oil

2 tablespoons rice vinegar

1 garlic clove, thinly sliced

1 teaspoon toasted sesame oil

1 teaspoon honey

3 tablespoons avocado oil

2 heads broccoli, halved lengthwise, stalks trimmed and peeled

1 fresh red finger chile, stemmed and thinly sliced

1 teaspoon sesame seeds, for garnish

Gluten-Free

Dairy-Free

Paleo

Grain-Free

Time: 30 minutes

VEGETABLES

SWEET PLANTAINS (MADUROS)

Gluten-Free

Dairy-Free

Whole30

Paleo

Grain-Free

Sugar-Free

Time: 15 minutes

2 tablespoons
avocado oil

3 yellow or brown
ripe plantains, peeled
and cut on an angle
into 2-inch-thick
slices

Kosher salt

Bring home some green plantains, and chances are that one or more will turn yellow or brown as quickly as you can say "tostones." If this happens, keep calm and make *maduros*! Ripe plantains can be quickly fried in some hot oil (avocado oil is preferred for its high smoking point and neutral flavor, but coconut oil works, too) and served alongside grilled meats or seafood. I particularly love them alongside my Jerk Chicken (page 55) because the sweetness balances the spice from the Scotch bonnet chiles in the Jerk Rub (page 257).

In a large nonstick skillet, heat the avocado oil over medium-high heat. Add the plantains and cook until browned on the bottom, 3 to 4 minutes. Flip and cook until golden brown on the second side, 3 to 4 minutes more.

Transfer to a plate and season with salt. Serve immediately.

GARLICKY RAPINI

Rapini, also referred to as broccoli rabe, is broccoli's slightly more aggressive cousin. It's bitter, peppery, and even more of an acquired taste, especially for kids. It should not be confused with Broccolini or tender-stem broccoli, the latter of which is a cross between Chinese broccoli (*gai lan*) and regular broccoli. To mellow the bitterness of the rapini, you can blanch it in a pot of salted boiling water before sautéing. This step has the added benefit of making the vegetable a bit more tender and really bringing out its dark-green color, which you will then set by shocking it in ice water. If you're living your Food Freedom or want to wow the in-laws at your next holiday dinner, try grating some aged hard Italian cheese over the top. You can't go wrong with Parmigiano Reggiano or Grana Padano.

This makes for a great side dish alongside my Mama's Roast Chicken (page 69), Emergency Roast Chicken (page 64), or Short Rib Ragù (page 103).

Fill a large bowl with ice and water and set it nearby.

Bring a large saucepan of water to a boil over high heat. Season the water with 1 tablespoon salt, add the rapini, and cook until the rapini is just tender but still crisp, 2 to 3 minutes. Transfer the rapini to the ice water and let sit until cool, 3 to 4 minutes, then drain fully in a colander. You can also gently squeeze the rapini to speed up the draining process but be careful not to break the florets.

While the rapini drains, in a large nonstick skillet, combine the olive oil and garlic. Cook gently over medium-low heat, stirring, until fragrant, 2 to 3 minutes. Add the red chile and cook, stirring, for 1 minute more. Add the rapini and cook, tossing occasionally, until everything is warmed through, about 2 minutes. Taste and season with salt.

Transfer the rapini to a platter. Garnish with the cheese, if desired, and serve with the lemon wedges alongside.

Kosher salt

1 pound rapini (broccoli rabe), tough stem ends trimmed but otherwise left whole

2 tablespoons extra-virgin olive oil

2 garlic cloves, thinly sliced

1 red finger chile, thinly sliced, or 1 teaspoon red pepper flakes

¼ cup grated Parmigiano Reggiano or Grana Padano cheese, for serving (optional)

½ lemon, cut into wedges, for serving

Gluten-Free

Dairy-Free

Whole30

Keto-Friendly

Paleo

Grain-Free

Sugar-Free

Time: 30 minutes

PATATAS BRAVAS

Gluten-Free

Dairy-Free

Whole30

Grain-Free

Sugar-Free

Time: 40 minutes

2 pounds white or yellow new or baby potatoes (about 1½ inches thick), halved

3 tablespoons avocado oil

½ teaspoon kosher salt, plus more if needed

¼ teaspoon freshly ground black pepper, plus more if needed

¼ cup Uncle Ronny's Romesco (page 243)

¼ cup Bootleg Garlic Sauce (page 234)

2 tablespoons finely chopped fresh chives, for garnish

Patatas bravas is a very common tapa (small shared dish) found throughout Spain. It's usually made with deep-fried chunks of potato smothered in a spicy tomato sauce. Sometimes it's also drizzled with a simple aioli, but things can get pretty creative, depending on the restaurant.

I travel to Spain often for research (I specialize in the early medieval architectural history of Asturias, an autonomous region in the northwest of the country), and the food is always something I look forward to. I've eaten my weight in *patatas bravas* over the years, and I really wanted to create a version that was easy enough to make on a weeknight but didn't sacrifice any of the flavor of the original. This one is pretty killer and delivers on all levels. I roast new potatoes (which I prefer for their shape and texture) and dot them with my romesco and Bootleg Garlic Sauce for an amazing interplay of flavors.

Preheat the oven to 425°F. Line a baking sheet with parchment paper.

In a large bowl, combine the potatoes, avocado oil, salt, and pepper and toss to coat. Arrange the potatoes in a single layer, cut-side down, on the prepared baking sheet. Roast for 30 to 35 minutes, until the potatoes are golden brown and tender. Check the potatoes halfway through the cooking time—you don't need to flip them as they cook, but if you do notice them cooking unevenly, rotate the baking sheet 180 degrees.

Carefully taste a potato and adjust the seasoning, if needed. Transfer the warm potatoes to a serving bowl and spoon the romesco and garlic sauce over the top. Garnish with the chives and serve immediately.

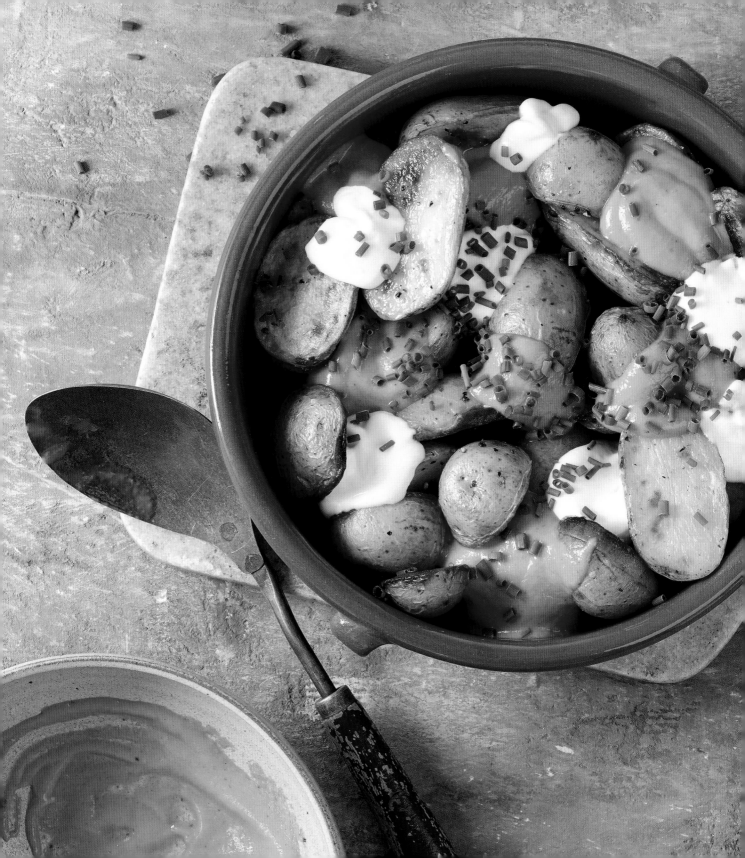

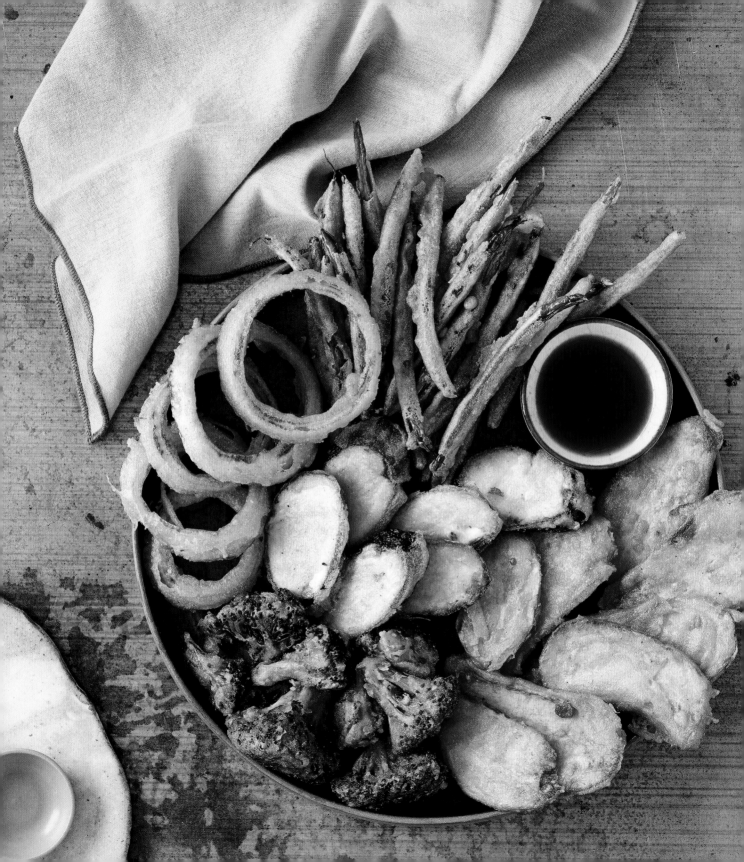

VEGETABLE TEMPURA

To make this vegetable tempura, I modify my Miracle Batter slightly, but as with my Miracle Fish and Chips (page 178) and Rock Shrimp (page 181), you'll never know the batter is gluten-free, grain-free, and Paleo. I've included some vegetable suggestions, but feel free to experiment with any you like. For me, nothing beats sweet potato tempura. Broccoli, green beans, and onion are all close seconds. Asparagus, on the other hand, was a disappointment during testing, though if you love asparagus you could give it a shot.

In a large nonstick skillet, heat the avocado oil over medium heat to 350°F. Line a plate with paper towels and place it near your frying station.

Working in batches, dredge the vegetables in the batter and gently shake off any excess. Carefully lay the vegetables in the hot oil and cook until golden brown, crispy, and cooked through, 3 to 4 minutes per side. Use a slotted spoon to transfer the vegetables to the paper towels to absorb excess oil. Repeat to batter and fry the remaining vegetables.

Sprinkle with salt while they're hot and serve with the coconut aminos alongside for dipping.

½ cup avocado oil, plus more if needed

1 sweet potato, thinly sliced on an angle

1 zucchini, thinly sliced on an angle

1 large yellow onion, sliced into ½-inch-thick rings

2 cups broccoli florets

4 ounces fresh green beans (about 1 cup)

½ cup Miracle Batter (page 247; omit the paprika and granulated onion)

Kosher salt

¼ cup coconut aminos, for dipping

Gluten-Free
Dairy-Free
Paleo
Grain-Free
Sugar-Free

Time: 35 minutes

BROCCOLI "CHEDDAR" SOUP

Gluten-Free

Dairy-Free

Whole30

Paleo

Grain-Free

Sugar-Free

Time: 45 minutes

2 tablespoons extra-virgin olive oil

1 yellow onion, diced

1 carrot, diced

Kosher salt and freshly ground black pepper

2 garlic cloves, coarsely chopped

1 teaspoon sweet paprika

½ teaspoon cayenne pepper (optional)

4 cups chicken stock

3 small sweet potatoes, peeled and cut into 2-inch cubes (about 3½ cups)

2 heads broccoli (about 1½ pounds), finely chopped, including stems

¼ cup nutritional yeast powder or flakes

A Paleo and Whole30-compliant broccoli "cheddar" soup? Could such a thing exist? Well, there's actually no cheddar in the soup, but there's a whole lotta cheesy flavor thanks to the addition of nutritional yeast. Serve it up as is, or take things to the next level by topping it with some of Catalina's Ground Meat Taco filling (page 114) and garnishing with it fresh cilantro and thinly sliced scallions. If that's not epic enough, go ahead and serve it with some Cassava Flour Tortillas (page 226) for dipping. If this soup doesn't get your kids to eat broccoli, I don't know what will!

In a large Dutch oven or heavy-bottomed pot, heat the olive oil over medium-high heat. Add the onion and carrot and season with ¼ teaspoon each salt and black pepper. Cook, stirring, until the vegetables are slightly softened, 5 to 6 minutes. Add the garlic and cook, stirring, for an additional minute, followed by the paprika and cayenne (if using), and cook, stirring, for 1 minute more so everything is evenly coated with the spices.

Add the stock, sweet potatoes, and all but 1½ cups of the broccoli. Add 4 cups water and bring to a boil. Cook at a boil until the sweet potatoes are fork-tender, about 12 minutes. Stir in the nutritional yeast. Remove from the heat and use an immersion blender to blend the soup until smooth and creamy. (Alternatively, let the soup cool slightly, carefully transfer it to a blender, and blend until smooth and creamy, then return the soup to the pot.) Taste and adjust the salt and pepper, as desired.

Stir in the remaining florets and cook over medium heat until the broccoli is just tender, 2 to 3 minutes. Let the soup cool for 5 to 10 minutes, then ladle it into individual bowls and serve.

Note: Did you know that broccoli stems are edible and delicious? Simply trim off the very bottom of the stem and use a vegetable peeler to peel off the tough outer layer, then chop the stem and add it to the soup. Or reserve the stems to use in a stir-fry.

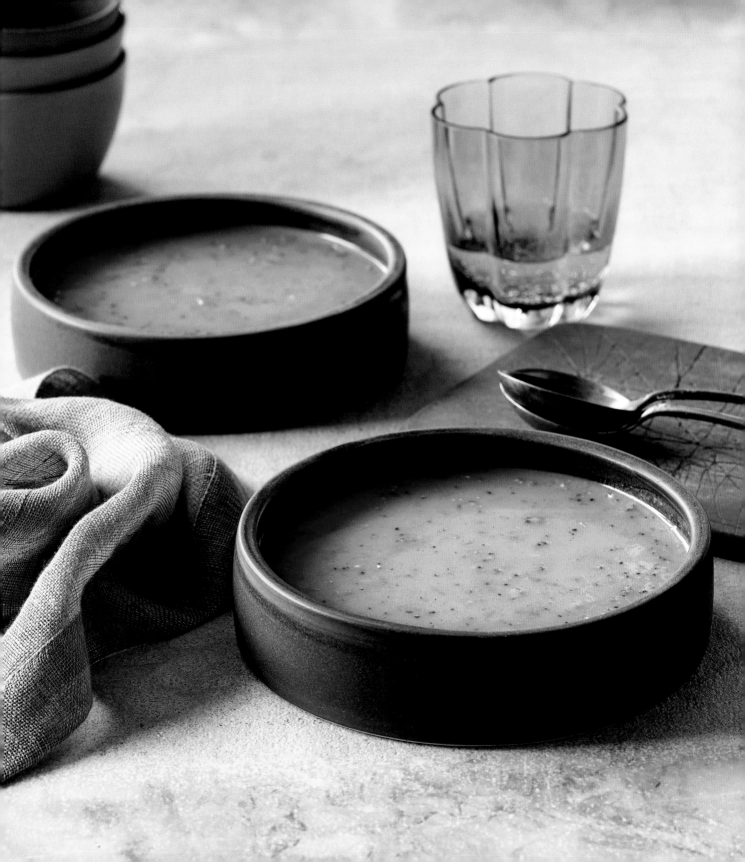

TWICE-FRIED PLANTAINS

Gluten-Free

Dairy-Free

Whole30

Paleo

Grain-Free

Sugar-Free

Time: 35 minutes

½ cup avocado oil, plus more as needed

3 large green plantains, peeled and cut on an angle into ½-inch-thick discs

Flaky sea salt

Tostones, patacones, tachinos, chatinos, tajadas, twice-fried plantains—no matter what you call them, these delicious crispy discs of heavenly goodness are hard to beat. (But for the sake of convenience, I'll refer to them as "tostones" from here on out.) Tostones are made with unripened green plantains and are fried twice, as opposed to *maduros* (see page 210), which are made with yellow or brown ripe plantains and are fried just once.

Everyone and their *abuela* has an opinion when it comes to frying tostones, and as a Russian-Jewish kid who grew up in Toronto, I'm not sure mine qualifies, at least not in any authoritative manner. What I can share with you, however, are a few tips I've picked up from frying my weight in green plantains.

1. Tostones are only made with green plantains. The green color refers to the skin of the fruit, not its flesh, and green skin means the plantain is unripened and firm. (If your plantains are yellow, brown, or almost black, use them for maduros, an absolutely divine but altogether different dish.)

2. Tostones are double-fried. You must first lightly fry or blanch the plantains in hot oil, remove them, and smash them before sending them back to the skillet for a second oil bath. This is a very necessary step that you cannot skip.

3. Use a high-smoking-point oil, such as coconut oil or avocado oil. Avocado oil is my preference; it has a high smoking point and is neutral in flavor. Coconut oil will add a slight coconut flavor to your tostones.

4. You can shallow-fry or deep-fry the tostones, but the latter method will require more oil, all of which you'll likely discard after frying. This can get expensive if you're using avocado oil, so I don't advise deep-frying. Instead, grab a nonstick skillet and shallow-fry the plantains. Unlike cast iron, nonstick skillets won't absorb any oil as you cook. For shallow-frying, use enough oil to come at

least halfway up the side of the plantains. Some of the oil will be absorbed by the plantains in each batch, so be sure to keep an eye on the oil level and add more as needed between batches, or the tostones will scorch.

5. Go as thin or thick as you like. There are those who will argue tooth and nail that tostones are not tostones unless they are thick, dense, and deeply browned. Others prefer a thinner, crispier, golden brown finished product. I have come realize that different cultures approach the dish differently, and a specific region, town, or family will have even more opinions.

6. You can soak the tostones in vinegar and/or adobo. My friend José and his lovely wife, Maria, both from Venezuela, invited Catalina and me over for dinner one night and made us their tostones. They were, by no stretch of the imagination, magical! The secret? After the first round of frying, José soaked the plantains in a bowl of distilled white vinegar mixed with adobo seasoning. Not only does this infuse the plantains with an insane amount of flavor, but it causes a reaction between the liquid and the hot oil during the second round of frying, which makes the plantains even crispier. You can also dip the plantains in water after the first round of frying to get a similar effect.

In a 10-inch nonstick skillet, heat ¼ cup of the avocado oil over medium-high heat to 350°F. Line a baking sheet with paper towels and place it near your frying station.

Working in batches, if needed, carefully lay the plantains in the hot oil and fry until golden, 2 to 3 minutes per side. Transfer the par-cooked plantains to the baking sheet and repeat to fry the remaining plantains, adding more oil as needed.

recipe continues

One at a time, place the plantain slices between two sheets of waxed paper and gently smash them to ½ inch thick using a flat-bottomed cup, ramekin, or tortilla press.

Bring the oil back to 350°F. Again working in batches, carefully lay the smashed plantains in the hot oil and fry until golden brown and crispy, 2 to 3 minutes per side. Add more oil to the pan as needed. Transfer the tostones to the baking sheet and season with flaky salt. Serve immediately.

NACHO-CHEESY CASHEWS

Careful, these spiced cashews are dangerously addictive! They're a bit spicy and taste nacho-cheesy thanks to the nutritional yeast, which is Whole30- and Paleo-compliant. Look for nutritional yeast that comes in powder form, because it will stick to the nuts a bit better than nutritional yeast flakes. If you can't find nutritional yeast powder, though, go ahead and use the flakes.

In a dry nonstick skillet, toast the cashews over medium-low heat, stirring occasionally, until warm, about 4 minutes. Add the avocado oil, toss to coat the nuts, and cook, stirring occasionally, until the cashews are golden, 2 to 3 minutes more. Add the nutritional yeast, paprika, flaky salt, and cayenne and toss to coat. Taste the nuts for seasoning and adjust the salt and cayenne pepper as desired.

Transfer the nuts to a serving dish. Let cool for at least 5 minutes before serving. Store in an airtight container at room temperature for up to 1 week.

1 cup raw unsalted cashews

1 tablespoon avocado oil

1 tablespoon nutritional yeast powder or flakes

1 teaspoon sweet paprika

1 teaspoon flaky sea salt

⅛ teaspoon cayenne pepper, plus more to taste

Gluten-Free

Dairy-Free

Whole30

Keto-Friendly

Paleo

Grain-Free

Time: 15 minutes

CREAMY HUMMUS
WITH SPICED CHICKPEAS

Gluten-Free
Dairy-Free
Grain-Free
Sugar-Free

Time: 30 minutes,
plus at least
1 hour of
refrigeration

**For the Creamy
Hummus:**

1 (15.5-ounce) can
chickpeas, drained

¼ cup tahini

2 tablespoons fresh
lemon juice, plus
more as needed

1 garlic clove, finely
chopped

1 teaspoon kosher
salt, plus more as
needed

¼ cup ice water

**For the Spiced
Chickpeas:**

3 tablespoons extra-
virgin olive oil

1 onion, diced

2 garlic cloves, finely
chopped

1 teaspoon ground
cumin

1 teaspoon ground
coriander

1 teaspoon sweet
paprika

¾ teaspoon kosher
salt

½ teaspoon ground
turmeric

½ teaspoon cayenne
pepper

Let's face it—hummus is the stuff of legends. Even people who hate vegetables are 99.9 percent more likely to grab some raw celery, broccoli, or cauliflower just so they can dunk it in creamy, garlicky, delicious hummus.

I realize that hummus is made with chickpeas, a legume, and is, therefore, neither Paleo nor Whole30-compliant. However, if you find you tolerate chickpeas well, a homemade chickpea spread is a great option to incorporate into your Food Freedom. Making it from scratch is not only easy, it's also more affordable than buying prepared hummus from the store, and it allows you to control the ingredients.

Personally, I have no problem enjoying hummus in moderation, and this particular version, topped with spiced chickpeas, is a family favorite. It's become one of my signature appetizers at holiday gatherings, and it's usually the first thing on the table to be devoured. It's super easy and flavorful. For the sake of convenience, I use canned chickpeas, but you could cook dried chickpeas and use those instead, if you prefer. Soak dried chickpeas in water overnight before boiling them in some baking soda–spiked water. Aside from that, the recipe is the same.

The secret to a super-creamy hummus is to remove the skin from each chickpea. As tedious as this is, the result is a much silkier finished product, so I encourage you to give it a try at least once, if you have the time. It isn't a mandatory step, though, so don't worry too much about skipping it if you're rushing to get dinner on the table before your in-laws arrive.

For me, the star of the show is actually the spiced chickpeas that get spooned over the hummus, rather than the hummus itself. This move is inspired by *hummus masabacha*, in which whole chickpeas are used as garnish over a bed of hummus. It's incredibly delicious and is just as great as a side dish for lean protein or over Cauliflower Rice (page 205) or steamed rice, if it's part of your Food Freedom.

MAKE THE CREAMY HUMMUS: Fill a large bowl with cold water and add the chickpeas. Using your hands, gently rub the chickpeas together under the water to release their skins. Skim off and discard the skins as they rise to the surface.

Drain the chickpeas and transfer them to a food processor. Process until finely crumbled, then use a silicone spatula to scrape down the sides of the bowl. With the motor running, add the tahini, lemon juice, garlic, and salt and process until a paste forms, about 1 minute. Scrape down the sides of the bowl once again. With the motor running, slowly add the ice water, then process until the mixture is smooth and creamy, 4 to 5 minutes, stopping to scrape down the sides of the bowl every minute or so.

Taste and season with more salt and lemon juice as desired. Transfer the hummus to a bowl, cover, and refrigerate for at least 1 hour before serving. (The hummus can be stored in the refrigerator for up to 1 week.)

MAKE THE SPICED CHICKPEAS: In a large nonstick or stainless-steel skillet, heat the olive oil over medium heat. Add the onion and cook, stirring, until softened and slightly caramelized, 8 to 10 minutes. Add the garlic and cook, stirring, for 1 minute. Stir in the cumin, coriander, paprika, salt, turmeric, and cayenne and cook, stirring often, for another minute. Add the chickpeas and toss to coat.

Pour in the stock and bring the mixture to a gentle simmer. Cook until the liquid has reduced by about half, 8 to 10 minutes.

Spread the hummus over the bottom of a shallow serving bowl and use a large spoon to make a well in the center. Pour the spiced chickpeas into the well and garnish with the parsley. Serve immediately.

1 (15.5-ounce) can chickpeas, drained and rinsed

1 cup chicken stock or water

3 fresh parsley leaves, for garnish

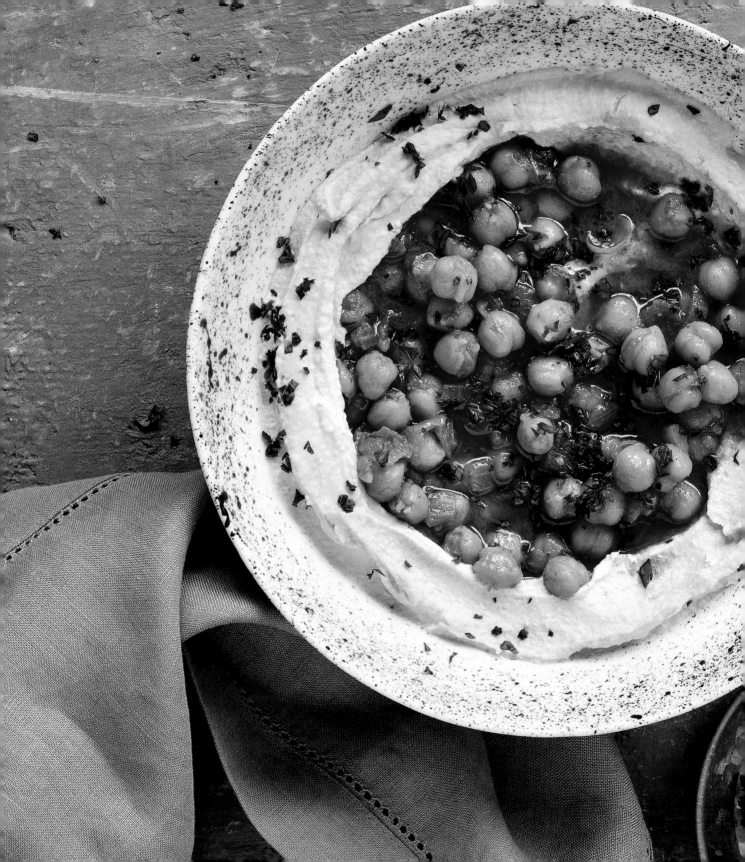

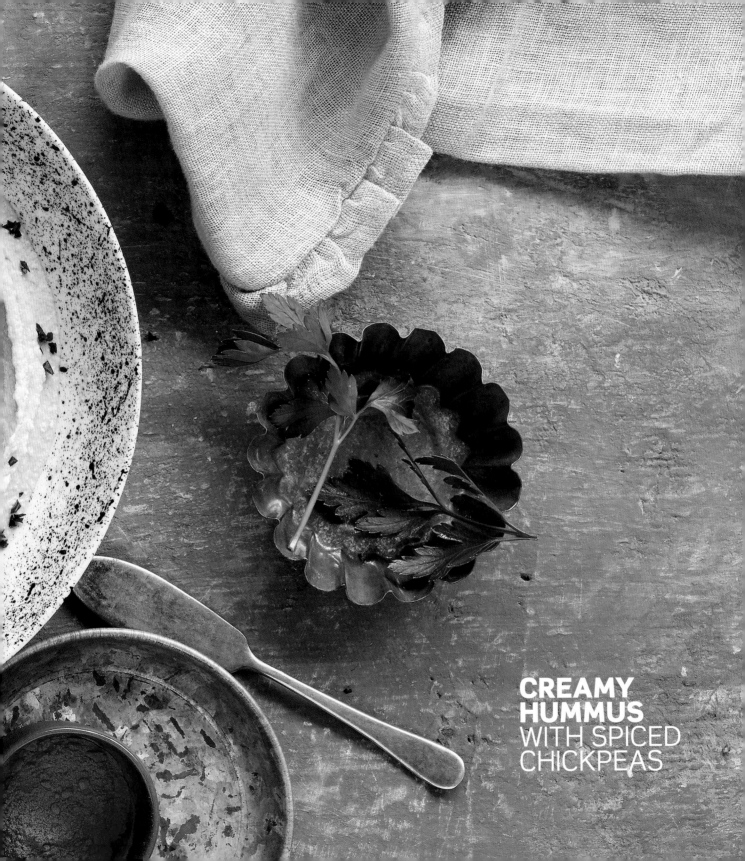

CREAMY
HUMMUS
WITH SPICED
CHICKPEAS

CASSAVA FLOUR TORTILLAS

Gluten-Free

Dairy-Free

Paleo

Grain-Free

Sugar-Free

Time: 30 minutes

1 cup cassava flour

2 tablespoons avocado oil

¼ teaspoon fine sea salt

¼ teaspoon baking soda

⅔ cup warm water

Though these tortillas are made with Whole30-compliant ingredients, they would be considered SWYPO (see page xxii) and, therefore, are off-limits during your round of Whole30. They are, however, Paleo and would be a wonderful addition to your Food Freedom. Enjoy them with Catalina's Ground Meat Tacos (page 114), Tomatillo Beef Soup (page 119), Slow Cooker Mojo Pork (page 150), and Cochinita Pibil (page 143).

The tortilla dough could not be simpler to make and is surprisingly easy to handle. If your dough is too dry and cracks, add water a teaspoon at a time and work it into the dough. If the dough is too wet and sticks to the waxed paper, add more flour a teaspoon at a time. As I was testing this recipe, the amount of water required tended to vary, so I recommend measuring ⅔ cup water and adding it a little at a time, rather than all at once.

For best results, use a tortilla press lined with waxed paper. They're affordable and can be purchased online. Alternatively, you can use a flat-bottomed bowl, such as a glass food storage bowl, to press the dough flat. Be sure to do this on a sturdy surface and to place the dough between sheets of waxed paper to prevent sticking.

In a medium bowl, combine the cassava flour, avocado oil, salt, and baking soda and mix with your hands until crumbly; you want to coat as much of the flour with oil as possible.

While mixing with one hand, slowly stream in the warm water until you can form the dough into a ball. The dough should hold its shape but also be very moist. (You may not use all the water.)

Roll the dough into an 8-inch-long log and cut it crosswise into 8 equal pieces for smaller tortillas or 6 equal pieces for larger tortillas. Roll each piece into a ball and place them in a large bowl. Cover the bowl with a damp kitchen towel.

Heat a large nonstick or cast-iron skillet over medium-high heat. Line a 2-quart saucepan with a clean kitchen towel.

Set a sheet of waxed paper or parchment paper on the bottom plate of a tortilla press. Place one ball of dough in the press and top it with another sheet of waxed paper. Flatten the ball of dough using the press. Remove the tortilla and carefully peel off the waxed paper. Place the tortilla in the hot skillet. Cook until golden on the bottom, 60 to 90 seconds, then flip and cook for 60 to 90 seconds on the second side. If you did it right, the tortilla will puff up ever so slightly; this is a good sign. If the tortilla does not puff up, try gently tapping on it with your fingertips while it is cooking (just be careful, as the pan is hot).

Transfer the cooked tortilla to the prepared pan and cover it gently with the edges of the towel to keep warm; cover with the lid. Repeat to form and cook the remaining tortillas. Serve immediately while still warm.

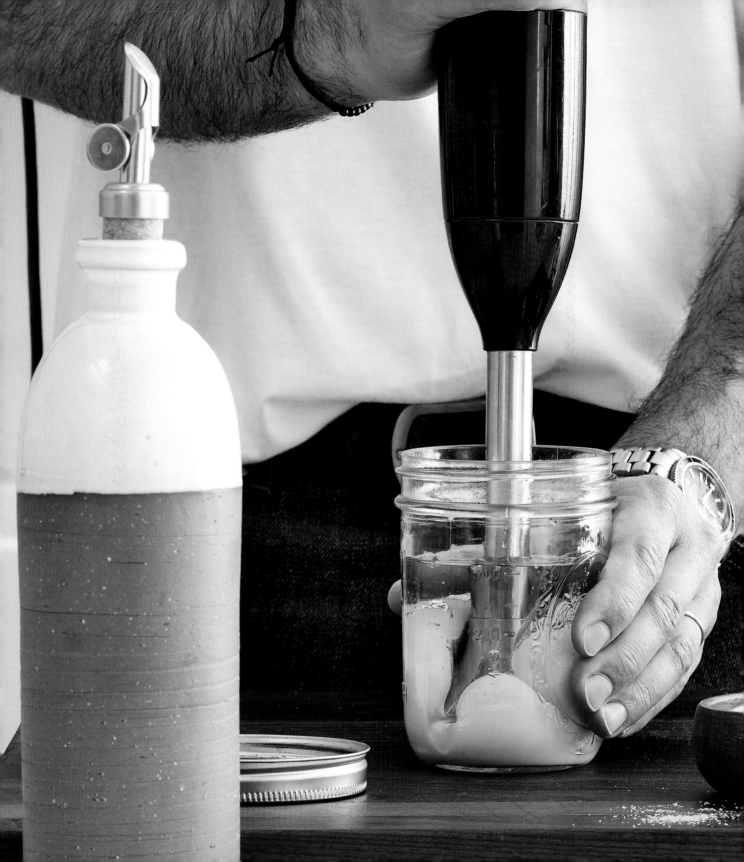

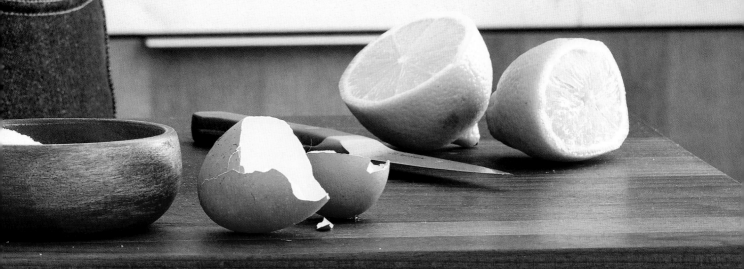

SAUCES, DRESSINGS, AND SPICE BLENDS

SAUCES

30-MISSISSIPPI MAYONNAISE

Gluten-Free

Dairy-Free

Whole30

Keto-Friendly

Paleo

Grain-Free

Time: 5 minutes, plus 1 hour of refrigeration

1 cup avocado oil

1 large egg, at room temperature

2 teaspoons fresh lemon juice

1 teaspoon Dijon mustard

Sea salt

It will take you a count of 30 Mississippis to make this Whole30- and Paleo-compliant mayonnaise. To minimize cleanup and waste, I make the mayo in a widemouthed mason jar that has units of measure right on the side. The mayo will keep for about 5 days in the refrigerator and is a key ingredient in my Bootleg Garlic Sauce (page 234), Caraway Cabbage Coleslaw (page 2), Creamy Fennel and Celery Slaw (page 5), Classic Deviled Eggs (page 20), and Rock Shrimp (page 181).

Refrain from using extra-virgin olive oil when making homemade mayonnaise. Its flavor is too strong and bitter. Avocado oil is my preferred oil because it is heart-healthy, light-colored, and neutral in flavor, and it's what I use in a great deal of my cooking, which means I usually have it in my pantry. I stock up on 1-quart bottles from Costco for a fraction of what it costs in regular grocery stores. If you absolutely cannot get your hands on avocado oil, then extra-light-flavored olive oil is your second best option. However, keep in mind that this is a highly refined oil that has had most of its nutrients stripped away.

In a widemouthed mason jar, combine the avocado oil, egg, lemon juice, and mustard. Center the head of the immersion blender over the egg yolk and blend on the lowest speed (if your blender has multiple speeds), without moving the blender, for a count of 15 Mississippis, until the bottom half of the oil is emulsified.

Slowly move the immersion blender up and down for an additional 15 Mississippis to gradually emulsify the remaining oil. Taste the mayonnaise and season with salt to taste (it likely won't take more than a pinch). Blend to combine. Cover the jar with a lid and refrigerate for at least 1 hour before using.

Notes: If making mayonnaise by hand, in a large bowl, whisk together the egg, lemon juice, and mustard to combine. While whisking, slowly drizzle in all the oil. Taste and add more salt as needed.

If your mayonnaise separates or "breaks," pour it into a large bowl, then, while vigorously whisking the separated mayonnaise, add a couple of drops of boiling water. The heat from the water should re-emulsify the mayonnaise.

BASIC GUACAMOLE

Gluten-Free

Dairy-Free

Whole30

Keto-Friendly

Paleo

Grain-Free

Sugar-Free

Time: 10 minutes

2 ripe avocados (see sidebar)

¼ cup finely chopped white onion

¼ cup finely chopped fresh cilantro leaves

Juice of 1 lime, plus more if needed

Kosher salt

Think of this basic guacamole as a starting point for a world of possibilities. Sure, it's good as is, but here are some ideas on how to take things to the next level, if you dare.

- Add a dash or two of Tajín, a tangy Mexican spice mixture that is Whole30-compliant.

- Add a finely chopped chipotle chile in adobo. Though most are packed with a small amount of sugar, and therefore are neither Paleo nor Whole30-compliant, the spice and smokiness from the pepper transforms the taste of your guac into something spectacular. The downside is that it will tint the guacamole slightly brown. But who cares? It's delicious!

- Add a dash of ground chipotle chile. Not nearly as flavorful as canned chipotles in adobo, but a great option for a Whole30- and Paleo-compliant alternative if you want to add some kick to your guac.

- Add some roasted garlic. You'll get an unexpected pop of sweet, caramelized, garlicky flavor that will have you coming back for more and more.

In a medium bowl, combine the avocados, onion, cilantro, lime juice, and a pinch of salt and stir until mostly smooth but still slightly chunky. Taste and adjust the seasoning with more salt or lime juice, as desired. Serve immediately.

HOW TO PICK A RIPE AVOCADO

1. Look for ones with the stems still intact. This prevents the inside from oxidizing (turning brown).
2. Remove the stem and look at the color beneath it. If it's a light green, the avocado is ripe. If it's brown, chances are the flesh inside is as well.
3. The skin should be almost black, not green, if you're using a Hass avocado.
4. It should be a little soft but with some spring to it. Test for softness near the stem so you don't bruise or misshape the center.

To ripen avocados overnight, place them in a paper bag with a banana. Bananas naturally give off a gas that speeds up the ripening process.

BOOTLEG GARLIC SAUCE

Gluten-Free

Dairy-Free

Whole30

Keto-Friendly

Paleo

Grain-Free

Sugar-Free

Time: 5 minutes

½ cup 30-Mississippi Mayonnaise (page 230)

2 tablespoons fresh lemon juice

2 teaspoons finely chopped garlic

I could drink this stuff by the glass! It's garlicky and lemony, and it tastes amazing on absolutely everything. It's a shortcut version of the Lebanese garlic sauce *toum* (see page 242), hence the "bootleg" in the title, but still packs a flavorful punch on things like Chicken Shawarma (page 52) and Patatas Bravas (page 212).

In a small bowl, combine the mayonnaise, lemon juice, and garlic and stir until fully combined. Cover and refrigerate until ready to serve. The sauce will keep in the refrigerator for up to 5 days.

CHA CHA CHIMICHURRI

Chimichurri is the ultimate summertime condiment, serving double duty as both a sauce and a marinade (see page 132). I always start my chimichurri by making a saltwater solution. It's something I originally saw Francis Mallmann do way back when, and I've riffed on it ever since. I prefer the taste and texture this way, as opposed to a purely oil-based sauce, like one of my salsa verdes (see pages 237 and 244). This is especially true when I serve chimichurri with rich, fatty cuts of meat, which don't necessarily need more oil.

In a medium bowl, combine the boiling water and the salt. Stir until the salt has dissolved, about 30 seconds, and let the water cool to room temperature. Add the parsley, cilantro, vinegar, olive oil, shallot, mint, garlic, oregano, red pepper flakes, and paprika and stir to combine. Transfer to a mason jar, cover, and refrigerate for up to 2 weeks. If you do refrigerate the sauce to use later, let it come to room temperature before serving, as the olive oil will have solidified a bit.

Note: You could make the whole thing right in the mason jar. The glass used to make canning jars is tempered, so the boiling water won't be an issue.

½ cup boiling water

1 teaspoon kosher salt

½ cup finely chopped fresh parsley leaves

½ cup finely chopped fresh cilantro leaves

¼ cup red wine vinegar

¼ cup extra-virgin olive oil

1 shallot, finely chopped

8 to 10 fresh mint leaves, finely chopped

1 garlic clove, finely chopped or mashed to a paste

1 teaspoon dried oregano

1 teaspoon red pepper flakes, or 1 fresh red chile, such as Anaheim or finger, finely chopped

1 teaspoon smoked Spanish paprika

Gluten-Free

Dairy-Free

Whole30

Paleo

Grain-Free

Sugar-Free

Keto-Friendly

Time: 10 minutes

CIVILAKE TIZAKI
(COCONUT TZATZIKI)

Gluten-Free

Dairy-Free

Whole30

Keto-Friendly

Paleo

Grain-Free

Time: 10 minutes,
plus 2 days
for coconut
fauxgurt

For the Coconut Fauxgurt:

1 (13.5-ounce) can full-fat coconut milk, refrigerated overnight

2 probiotic capsules (not pills or tablets)

For the Civilake Tizaki:

1 Persian cucumber, peeled, seeded, and finely chopped (about 2 tablespoons)

Grated zest and juice of ½ lemon

1 tablespoon finely chopped fresh parsley or dill

1 garlic clove, finely chopped

½ teaspoon dried oregano

1 teaspoon dried mint

1 teaspoon dried basil

Kosher salt and freshly ground black pepper

Tzatziki is a garlicky, lemony, and herbaceous Greek yogurt–based condiment. It's amazing with my Mama's Roast Chicken (page 69) or grilled meats and veggies. Here I replace the traditional dairy-based yogurt with "fauxgurt" made from thickened coconut cream and the contents of two probiotic capsules. To make the fauxgurt extra thick, I place an unshaken can of coconut milk in the refrigerator overnight so that the cream solidifies and rises to the top. For a thinner version, feel free to use the entire contents of a can of full-fat coconut milk.

The odd title for this sauce goes back to my childhood, when a friend of my brother's pronounced "souvlaki with tzatziki" as "civilake with tizaki." It's stuck with me ever since. (His name is Drew Engel. He was a freestyle Rollerblader. Do people still Rollerblade? It was big in the '90s.)

MAKE THE COCONUT FAUXGURT: Without shaking the can, carefully open it and spoon 1 cup of the solidified white cream into a mason jar (save any remaining coconut cream and the coconut water left in the can for another use). Add the contents of the probiotic capsules to the jar and stir together with a nonreactive spoon (such as one made from plastic or wood). Cover the jar with cheesecloth and let stand at room temperature for 48 hours, until slightly thickened. Transfer the fauxgurt to the refrigerator until ready to use. (It will keep in the refrigerator for up to 5 days.)

MAKE THE CIVILAKE TIZAKI: In a medium bowl, combine 1 cup of the coconut fauxgurt, the cucumber, lemon zest, lemon juice, parsley, garlic, oregano, mint, and basil. Mix until well combined. Taste and adjust the salt, pepper, and lemon juice as needed. Cover and refrigerate for at least 1 hour before serving to allow the flavors to come together. Store any leftovers in the refrigerator for up to 5 days.

CLASSIC SALSA VERDE

I am of the firm opinion that this salsa verde tastes best when made by hand. You just can't beat the texture of the finely chopped herbs, garlic, and anchovies. However, as a new dad, I realize now, more than ever before, that time is of the essence! So I am, somewhat reluctantly, including a food-processor method. Just keep in mind that the food processor will either turn your salsa into a puree (not a good thing here) or leave some pieces larger than others (also not a good thing). If you want to err on the side of caution and go the old-fashioned route, simply finely chop all the ingredients and combine them in a bowl.

I know what you're thinking, and yes, the anchovies are necessary here. Of course, there's nothing I can do to stop you from omitting them if you can't stomach them, but I encourage you to give them a try before you make up your mind. Without them and the capers, you might as well make Uncle Ronny's Salsa Verde (page 244).

Spoon this salsa over grilled steak, chicken, or pork, and be sure to try it with my Emergency Roast Chicken (page 64) for a homemade riff on Jonathan Waxman's famous JW Chicken!

2 olive oil–packed anchovy fillets

2 garlic cloves, peeled

1 tablespoon capers, drained

1 cup extra-virgin olive oil

1 cup loosely packed fresh parsley, coarsely chopped

¼ cup loosely packed fresh basil leaves, torn by hand

1 jalapeño, seeded (if you prefer less heat) and coarsely chopped

Juice of 1 lemon

Kosher salt and freshly ground black pepper

Gluten-Free

Dairy-Free

Whole30

Keto-Friendly

Paleo

Grain-Free

Sugar-Free

Time: 10 minutes

In a food processor, combine the anchovies, garlic, and capers and process to form a paste. Scrape down the sides of the bowl with a spatula and add the olive oil, parsley, basil, jalapeño, and lemon juice. Pulse until the salsa is chunky and just combined. Taste the salsa and season with salt and pepper as desired. Transfer the salsa to a jar, cover, and set aside at room temperature (for a maximum of 4 hours) until ready to serve. The salsa can be stored in the refrigerator for up to 5 days.

KALE AND WALNUT PESTO

Gluten-Free

Dairy-Free

Whole30

Keto-Friendly

Paleo

Grain-Free

Sugar-Free

Time: 20 minutes

1 pound lacinato kale (about 1 bunch)

Kosher salt and freshly ground black pepper

½ cup raw unsalted walnuts

1 garlic clove

1 tablespoon fresh lemon juice

½ cup extra-virgin olive oil

Try tossing this vibrant green pesto with crispy Roast Cauliflower (page 203) or, if you're living your Food Freedom, your favorite pasta, gluten-free or otherwise. I like to use lacinato kale (also known as cavolo nero, Tuscan kale, and dinosaur kale) and reserve the stems for my Kale Stem Frittata (page 37), but you can substitute regular curly kale if that's what you have on hand.

This pesto is especially great if you grow your own kale and find yourself with more than you know what to do with. Sadly, I've never had this problem because I am the world's worst gardener. If I did have this problem, I would make a big batch of this pesto, store it in mason jars, and freeze it to use throughout the winter.

Use your hands to strip the kale leaves from the stems.

Fill a large bowl halfway with cold water and add a couple of handfuls of ice. Set it nearby.

Bring a large saucepan of water to a boil. Season with 1 tablespoon salt, add the kale, and blanch for 3 minutes. Transfer the kale to the ice water and let cool completely, 3 to 4 minutes. Transfer the kale to a colander and squeeze it to drain well. Set aside.

In a small dry skillet, toast the walnuts over medium heat, stirring occasionally to prevent burning, until lightly browned and fragrant, about 3 minutes.

Transfer the walnuts to a food processor and add the kale, garlic, lemon juice, and a pinch each of salt and pepper. With the food processor running, slowly drizzle in the olive oil until fully incorporated. Taste and adjust the salt and pepper as desired.

Transfer the pesto to a jar, cover, and refrigerate until ready to use. The pesto will keep in the refrigerator for up to 5 days or in the freezer for up to 6 months.

PAPA'S HERBY KETCHUP

My father used to make this sauce once a week. He'd slather brown bread with butter, spoon this sauce over the top, and devour it with a look of sheer joy on his face. He'd also use it as a kind of ketchup for all kinds of grilled meats, particularly his Pan-Fried Lamb Chops (page 146).

I warn you, it packs a punch, especially for those who have a garlic sensitivity. It's loaded with fresh herbs (what my father calls "green stuff"), plenty of raw garlic, two types of onion, hot chile, lemon juice, tomato puree, fresh tomatoes, and oil. The only thing that's changed from his original recipe is my use of extra-virgin olive oil instead of sunflower oil. Oh, and I've also reduced the amount of garlic my father would use by half! The good news is, the flavors will mellow out and come together over time. In fact, this sauce tastes best the next day, making it great for times when you need to prep things ahead.

In a large bowl, combine the grated tomatoes, dill, parsley, cilantro, onion, tomato puree, oil, scallions, garlic, chile, lemon juice, and salt. Cover and let stand at room temperature for at least 30 minutes before serving. Store in the refrigerator in a sealable jar for up to 5 days.

½ cup grated fresh vine-ripened tomatoes (about 1 large)

½ cup loosely packed fresh dill, finely chopped

½ cup loosely packed fresh parsley leaves, finely chopped

½ cup loosely packed fresh cilantro leaves, finely chopped

½ cup finely chopped sweet white onion (see Note)

½ cup tomato puree (see Note)

¼ cup extra-virgin olive oil

2 scallions, white and light green parts only, finely chopped

2 garlic cloves, finely chopped

1 fresh red finger chile, seeded and finely chopped

1 tablespoon fresh lemon juice

1 teaspoon kosher salt

Gluten-Free

Dairy-Free

Whole30

Paleo

Grain-Free

Sugar-Free

Time: 15 minutes, plus 30 minutes of refrigeration

Notes: If you don't have sweet white onion, rinse chopped yellow onion under running water to mellow its flavor and use that instead.

If you can find something called tomato passata, use that instead of tomato puree. Tomato passata is most often sold in tall, narrow glass jars in the tomato sauce or pasta aisle of the grocery store. Sometimes you can find it in tetrapaks. Look for a passata that is made with nothing more than pureed and strained tomatoes and salt. If you can't find passata, and as an alternative to puree, I recommend combining 2 tablespoons tomato paste with ½ cup water. The flavor will be a bit more intense, but it will work if you're in a pinch.

TAHINI SAUCE

Gluten-Free
Dairy-Free
Whole30
Keto-Friendly
Paleo
Grain-Free
Sugar-Free

Time: 5 minutes

½ cup tahini (sesame seed paste)

1 tablespoon fresh lemon juice, plus more if needed

1 garlic clove, finely chopped

¼ teaspoon kosher salt, plus more if needed

½ cup very cold water

Tahini sauce is one of the most forgiving sauces you could ever hope to make. It's virtually impossible to mess up and can always be adjusted if you do. If your tahini sauce is on the thick side, simply add a touch more water. If it's thinner than you'd like, add a bit more tahini. Same goes for the salt, garlic, and lemon juice, which can all be adjusted to taste. If you don't have a food processor, grab a large bowl and a whisk—it will turn out just as tasty.

To make the tahini sauce, I use 100% sesame seed paste, a product that is, rather confusingly, also called tahini. The paste can be found in Middle Eastern markets, major grocery stores, and health food stores (it's sometimes also labeled "sesame seed butter"). On its own, it's too thick, but when loosened into a sauce it can be drizzled over any number of dishes, including my Roast Short Ribs (page 92), Chicken Shawarma (page 52), Siniyeh Bitaheena (page 155), or Sabich Platter (page 28). It can even be used as a dressing for Chopped Salad (page 6).

Because tahini is very affordable and readily available in Toronto, I don't bother making it from scratch. If that's not the case for you, you can make it at home: In a dry skillet, toast 1 cup (or more) of white, hulled sesame seeds over medium-low heat until golden and warmed through. Let cool, then transfer the seeds to a food processor or high-speed blender and process, scraping down the sides of the bowl every so often, until ground into a paste, around 5 minutes. Use this paste in place of store-bought tahini to make tahini sauce or hummus, or anywhere else tahini is called for.

In a food processor, combine the tahini, lemon juice, garlic, and salt and process until well combined and crumbly, about 1 minute. Scrape down the sides of the bowl with a spatula. With the motor running, slowly pour in the water and process until fully incorporated. Scrape down the sides of the bowl again and process until smooth and creamy. Taste and adjust the seasoning, adding more salt or lemon juice, if desired. You may store in the refrigerator, covered, for up to 1 month.

TERIYAKI SAUCE

This Paleo and Whole30-compliant Asian-inspired sauce works perfectly with chicken, beef, pork, seafood, and vegetable stir-fries. Simply combine all the ingredients in a mason jar, shake it like it owes you money, and pour it into the pan with the protein and veggies.

In a mason jar, combine the coconut aminos, garlic, arrowroot starch, sesame oil, ginger, red pepper flakes, fish sauce, and ¼ cup water. Cover tightly with a lid and shake vigorously until completely smooth. Store in the refrigerator for up to 2 weeks.

¼ cup coconut aminos

1 tablespoon grated garlic (about 3 cloves)

1 tablespoon arrowroot starch

1 tablespoon toasted sesame oil

1 teaspoon grated fresh ginger

1 teaspoon red pepper flakes

½ teaspoon fish sauce

Gluten-Free

Dairy-Free

Whole30

Paleo

Grain-Free

Sugar-Free

Time: 5 minutes

THE DRACULA KILLER
(TOUM)

Gluten-Free
Dairy-Free
Whole30
Keto-Friendly
Paleo
Grain-Free

Time: 5 minutes

15 garlic cloves, peeled

¼ teaspoon kosher salt, plus more if needed

2 tablespoons fresh lemon juice

1½ cups avocado oil

If you're looking to up your condiment game for your next BBQ, consider making some *toum*. This Lebanese garlic sauce packs a serious punch and is as easy to make as it is delicious. It is commonly served with a variety of kebabs, grilled meats, and shawarma (see page 52). You can also try it alongside roasted veggies, sweet potatoes, or different types of squash. I affectionately call this miracle sauce "the Dracula Killer" due to its sheer potency. For a milder and quicker version, try my Bootleg Garlic Sauce (page 234).

For best results, you'll want to use a food processor, not a blender or immersion blender. During testing, I found that a larger surface around the blade allowed for a more gradual and forgiving emulsification process. Also important to note: You really want to exaggerate how slowly you pour in the lemon juice and oil. To prevent you from pouring them in too quickly, use a measuring cup with a spout, which allows for a slow drizzle.

In a food processor, combine the garlic and salt. Pulse for 30 seconds, then scrape down the sides of the bowl with a silicone spatula. Repeat until the garlic is finely chopped and begins to form a paste, about 2 minutes.

With the food processor running (on the lowest setting, if yours comes with varying speeds), slowly drizzle in 1 tablespoon of the lemon juice. Once the lemon juice has been incorporated, slowly drizzle in ¾ cup of the oil. Stop the food processor, scrape down the sides of the bowl again, and repeat with the remaining lemon juice and oil. It is very important not to rush this process or your toum will separate.

Taste and season with additional salt, if desired. Transfer the toum to a jar, seal, and refrigerate for up to 1 month.

UNCLE RONNY'S ROMESCO

Romesco is a creamy and delicious sauce made with almonds and roasted red peppers. It's believed to have originated in northeast Spain as a condiment for seafood. In some ways, it's similar to other roasted red pepper sauces, like the Balkan *ajvar* or Romanian *zacuscă*. I've made it many times, both with and without the almonds, and love it either way. I've decided to exclude them here to make the sauce accessible to those who are allergic to nuts. It's still incredibly delicious without them, but feel free to add ¼ cup unsalted roasted almonds to the blender, if you desire.

Try serving the romesco with grilled meat, fish, and seafood. Or add a couple of fresh red chiles to the mix and use it as the hot sauce for my Patatas Bravas (page 212)!

Preheat the oven to 425°F.

In a large bowl, combine the bell peppers, onion, garlic, and oregano. Add 2 tablespoons of the olive oil and toss to coat. Season with salt and black pepper, toss once more, and spread the mixture evenly over a rimmed baking sheet. Roast for 30 to 35 minutes, until the vegetables are slightly caramelized.

Carefully transfer the roasted vegetables and any pan juices to a blender. Add the vinegar and blend on low speed until the mixture is smooth and creamy. Increase the blender speed to high and, with the blender running, slowly drizzle in the remaining 2 tablespoons olive oil. Taste and adjust the salt and pepper as desired.

Transfer the sauce to a jar, cover, and refrigerate for 30 minutes to 1 hour before serving. The romesco will keep in the refrigerator for up to 5 days or in the freezer for up to 6 months.

2 large red bell peppers, sliced into 1-inch-wide strips

1 red onion, sliced into 1-inch-wide strips

3 garlic cloves, smashed and peeled

1 tablespoon chopped fresh oregano leaves, or 1 teaspoon dried

4 tablespoons extra-virgin olive oil

Kosher salt and freshly ground black pepper

1 tablespoon sherry vinegar

Gluten-Free

Dairy-Free

Whole30

Paleo

Grain-Free

Sugar-Free

Time: 40 minutes, plus 30 minutes of refrigeration

UNCLE RONNY'S SALSA VERDE

Gluten-Free

Dairy-Free

Paleo

Grain-Free

Time: 10 minutes

1 cup loosely packed fresh cilantro, parsley, or a combination, finely chopped

½ cup avocado oil or extra-virgin olive oil

¼ cup finely chopped white onion

1 garlic clove, grated or minced

½ jalapeño, seeded (if you want less heat) and finely chopped

2 tablespoons fresh lemon juice

1 teaspoon pure maple syrup, agave nectar, or honey

Kosher salt and freshly ground black pepper

Spoon this salsa verde over grilled chicken, beef, pork, seafood, or vegetables. It's fresh, bright, and super easy to make. It's also wonderful with my Emergency Roast Chicken (page 64).

I like using avocado oil here because it's neutral in flavor and color, but feel free to substitute extra-virgin olive oil if that's what you have on hand. Even though I only use a teaspoon of maple syrup, agave, or honey in the salsa, that little bit goes a long way and completely transforms the sauce. Therefore, if you're doing a round of Whole30, I recommend making my Classic Salsa Verde (page 237), which is compliant, instead of omitting the natural sweetener here.

In a medium bowl, stir together the cilantro, avocado oil, onion, garlic, jalapeño, lemon juice, and maple syrup. Taste and season with salt and pepper. Cover and refrigerate until ready to serve. The salsa will keep in a sealed container in the refrigerator for up to 2 weeks, or in the freezer for up to 6 months.

WHOLE30 TARTAR SAUCE

To be enjoyed with Miracle Fish and Chips (page 178), Chicken Schnitzel (page 40), or just about anything else—it's that good!

In a medium bowl, whisk together the mayonnaise, dill, pickle, pickle juice, lemon juice, garlic, capers, mustard, and granulated onion until smooth. Taste and season with salt and pepper as desired. Cover and refrigerate the sauce for at least 30 minutes before serving to allow the flavors to come together. Refrigerate up to one week.

1 cup 30-Mississippi Mayonnaise (page 230)

¼ cup fresh dill, finely chopped

1 large sugar-free dill pickle, finely chopped (about ¼ cup)

2 tablespoons dill pickle juice (from the pickle jar)

2 tablespoons fresh lemon juice

1 garlic clove, finely chopped

1 tablespoon capers packed in brine, drained and finely chopped

1 tablespoon Dijon mustard

1 tablespoon granulated onion

Kosher salt and freshly ground black pepper

Gluten-Free

Dairy-Free

Whole30

Keto-Friendly

Paleo

Grain-Free

Sugar-Free

Time: 10 minutes, plus at least 30 minutes of chilling

SAUCES, DRESSINGS, AND SPICE BLENDS

ZHUG

Gluten-Free

Dairy-Free

Whole30

Keto-Friendly

Paleo

Grain-Free

Sugar-Free

Time: 5 minutes

4 jalapeños: 3 seeded, 1 left whole (for a little extra heat)

½ cup firmly packed fresh parsley leaves

½ cup firmly packed fresh cilantro leaves

½ cup extra-virgin olive oil

¼ cup fresh lemon juice

½ teaspoon ground cumin

½ teaspoon ground coriander

½ teaspoon kosher salt

Zhug is a fiery and herbaceous Yemeni sauce. It's used as a condiment on all varieties of pita sandwiches, on grilled meats like my Roast Short Ribs (page 92), or even on eggs like in my Sabich Platter (page 28).

Like all great sauces, everyone has their own version of *zhug*. Here I keep things very simple and accessible while preserving the fundamental flavors (and heat!) of common Yemeni versions. You can try experimenting with different proportions of spices and herbs or add dried fenugreek and/or caraway seeds. As long as you keep things spicy, you're on the right track! Otherwise, go ahead and make one of my salsa verdes (pages 237 and 244).

In a blender or food processor, combine the jalapeños, parsley, cilantro, olive oil, lemon juice, cumin, coriander, and salt. Pulse until the mixture is combined but not completely smooth. Transfer the mixture to a jar, cover, and refrigerate for up to 1 week.

Note: For less cleanup, try making this in a widemouthed mason jar using an immersion blender.

MIRACLE BATTER

There's a reason I refer to this as Miracle Batter. It's entirely grain-, gluten-, dairy-, and alcohol-free, yet sticks to nearly everything, gets super crispy, and tastes light and airy. Use it to make my Miracle Fish and Chips (page 178), Rock Shrimp (page 181), and Vegetable Tempura (page 215). For best results, only make the batter immediately before using it. Otherwise, the bubbles in the carbonated water will fizzle out and it won't have quite the same effect. If using flat water, you can make the batter up to one hour in advance, cover, and store it in the refrigerator so it stays cold.

Technically, the ingredients are Whole30-compliant. However, since you'll be using the batter to re-create indulgent foods, it goes against the rules of the program. Instead, keep it for your Food Freedom.

Sift the cassava flour, arrowroot starch, and baking powder into a large bowl. Add the salt, paprika, and onion powder and whisk to combine. Add the sparkling water and whisk until smooth. The mixture should have the consistency of pancake batter. If the batter is too thick, add more sparkling water 1 tablespoon at a time. If the batter is too wet, add more cassava flour 1 tablespoon at a time. Use immediately.

1 cup cassava flour, plus more if needed

2 tablespoons arrowroot starch

½ teaspoon baking powder

1 teaspoon kosher salt

1 teaspoon sweet paprika

1 teaspoon granulated onion

1⅓ cups ice-cold sparkling water, plus more if needed

Gluten-Free
Dairy-Free
Paleo
Grain-Free
Sugar-Free

Time: 5 minutes

DRESSINGS

CALIFORNIA CLASSIC
(BALSAMIC VINAIGRETTE)

Gluten-Free
Dairy-Free
Paleo
Grain-Free

Time: 5 minutes

¼ cup extra-virgin olive oil

2 tablespoons balsamic vinegar

1 teaspoon honey (omit for Whole30)

1 teaspoon Dijon mustard

1 garlic clove, finely grated

⅛ teaspoon kosher salt

⅛ teaspoon freshly ground black pepper

You can't go wrong with a classic balsamic vinaigrette. Drizzle it over just about any salad, especially my Grilled Shrimp Cobb (page 12). For a trip to the West Coast, try it with some mixed field greens, cucumbers, tomatoes, thinly sliced red onion, avocado, fresh strawberries, toasted pecans, and, if you're living your Food Freedom, goat cheese.

In a small bowl, whisk together the olive oil, vinegar, honey, mustard, garlic, salt, and pepper until emulsified. Use immediately or transfer to a jar, cover, and store in the refrigerator for up to 2 weeks.

CILANTRO-LIME VINAIGRETTE

Bright, fresh, herbaceous, and super flavorful, this cilantro vinaigrette elevates the blandest of lettuces. That's right, I'm talking to you, romaine!

In a blender or food processor, combine the cilantro, lime juice, garlic, agave nectar, salt, pepper, and 2 tablespoons water and blend on high speed until smooth. With the motor running, slowly add the olive oil and blend until fully combined. Use immediately or transfer to a jar, cover, and store in the refrigerator for up to 5 days.

¼ cup loosely packed fresh cilantro leaves

Juice of 1 lime

1 garlic clove

1 teaspoon agave nectar or honey (omit for Whole30)

¼ teaspoon kosher salt

¼ teaspoon freshly ground black pepper

¼ cup extra-virgin olive oil or avocado oil

Gluten-Free

Dairy-Free

Paleo

Grain-Free

Time: 5 minutes

Note: For less cleanup, try making this in a widemouthed mason jar using an immersion blender.

SAUCES, DRESSINGS, AND SPICE BLENDS

MAMBO ITALIANO VINAIGRETTE

Gluten-Free
Dairy-Free
Whole30
Keto-Friendly
Paleo
Grain-Free
Sugar-Free

Time: 5 minutes

½ cup extra-virgin olive oil

2 tablespoons red wine vinegar

2 tablespoons fresh lemon juice

1 teaspoon dried Italian seasoning

¼ teaspoon granulated onion

¼ teaspoon granulated garlic

¼ teaspoon kosher salt

¼ teaspoon freshly ground black pepper

This classic Italian vinaigrette is a great example of how just a few substitutions can transform a recipe. It's almost identical to my Big Fat Greek Dressing (see opposite) but uses red wine vinegar and dried Italian seasoning. Just like its Greek cousin, use this to dress salads or grilled meats, vegetables, and fish.

In a mason jar, combine the olive oil, vinegar, lemon juice, Italian seasoning, granulated onion, granulated garlic, salt, and pepper. Cover and shake vigorously until emulsified. Use immediately or store in the refrigerator for up to 2 weeks.

MY BIG FAT GREEK DRESSING

A Greek salad just isn't complete without a Greek vinaigrette. This one is not only super easy to make, it's also incredibly versatile. Pour it over salads or grilled meats, seafood or fish.

In a mason jar, combine the olive oil, lemon juice, vinegar, oregano, basil, mint, granulated garlic, salt, and pepper. Cover and shake vigorously until emulsified. Use immediately or store in the refrigerator for up to 2 weeks.

½ cup extra-virgin olive oil

2 tablespoons fresh lemon juice

2 tablespoons white wine vinegar

¼ teaspoon dried oregano

¼ teaspoon dried basil

¼ teaspoon dried mint

¼ teaspoon granulated garlic

¼ teaspoon kosher salt

¼ teaspoon freshly ground black pepper

Gluten-Free

Dairy-Free

Whole30

Keto-Friendly

Paleo

Grain-Free

Sugar-Free

Time: 5 minutes

MAY ALL YOUR PAIN BE CHAMPAGNE VINAIGRETTE

Gluten-Free

Dairy-Free

Paleo

Grain-Free

Time: 5 minutes

½ cup extra-virgin olive oil

2 tablespoons champagne vinegar

2 tablespoons fresh lemon juice

1 tablespoon finely chopped shallot

½ teaspoon finely chopped garlic

½ teaspoon Dijon mustard

½ teaspoon honey (omit for Whole30)

¼ teaspoon kosher salt

¼ teaspoon freshly ground black pepper

As simple and ubiquitous as a champagne vinaigrette may be, I think it's an important recipe to learn, not only because it allows you to experiment with the fat-to-acid ratio, but it also introduces beginner and intermediate home cooks to the big, wide world of vinegars! Let's face it—oils get all the attention, but vinegars often end up stealing the show. Not to mention the fact that champagne vinaigrette demands finely chopped fresh garlic and shallot, which is great for those who need to brush up on their knife skills.

In a mason jar, combine the olive oil, vinegar, lemon juice, shallot, garlic, mustard, honey, salt, and pepper. Cover and shake vigorously until emulsified. Use immediately or store in the refrigerator for up to 2 weeks.

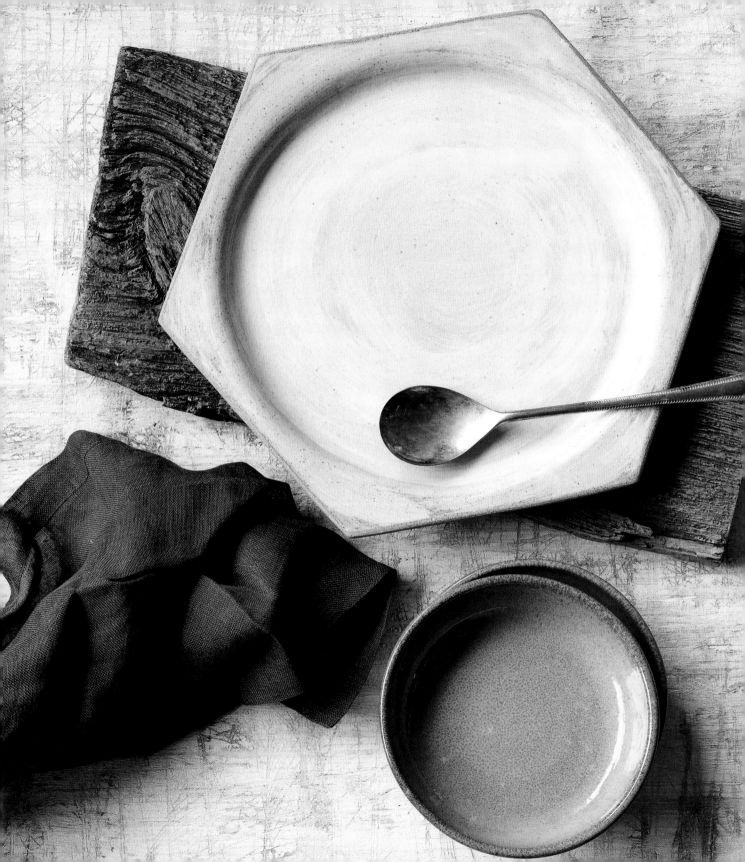

SPICE BLENDS

ADOBO SEASONING

Gluten-Free
Dairy-Free
Whole30
Keto-Friendly
Paleo
Grain-Free
Sugar-Free

Time: 5 minutes

1 tablespoon granulated onion

1 tablespoon granulated garlic

1 teaspoon dried oregano

1 teaspoon ground turmeric

1 teaspoon kosher salt

½ teaspoon freshly ground black pepper

My absolute favorite seasoning for all types of seafood, but especially shrimp! It's the flavor bomb behind my Grilled Shrimp Cobb (page 12), Steak Oscar (page 110), and Adobo Shrimp with Cauliflower "Grits" and Collard Greens (page 162). With this spice blend, and with all the others that follow, you can save time and reduce cleanup by making them in a mason jar. It's also a good idea to label and date each one so that you know what it is and how long it's good for.

In a small jar, combine all the ingredients. Seal the jar and shake to combine. Store in a cool, dry place for up to 1 month.

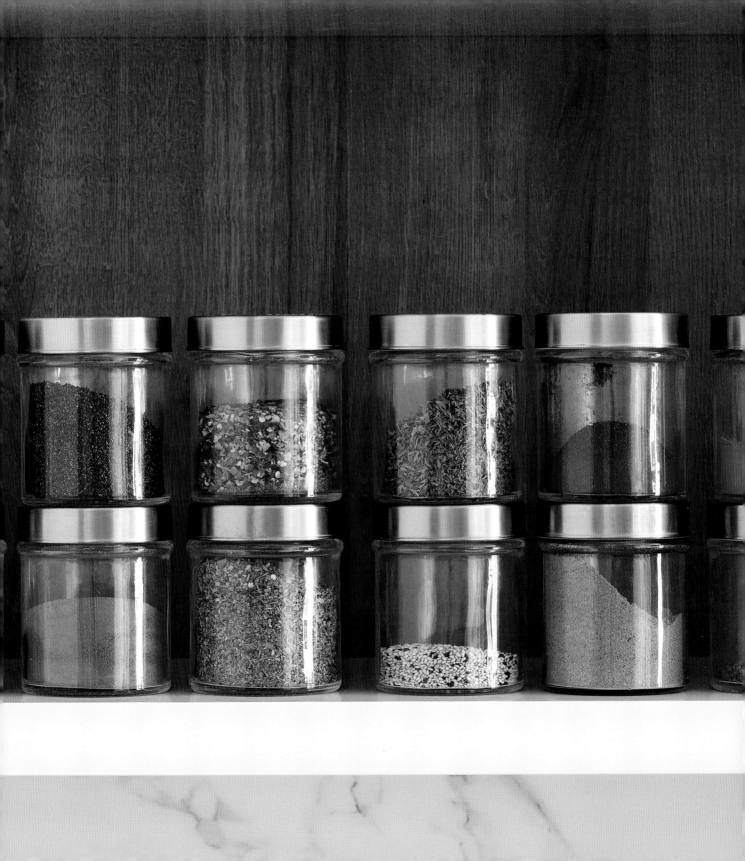

BAGEL BE GONE SEASONING

Gluten-Free

Dairy-Free

Whole30

Keto-Friendly

Paleo

Grain-Free

Sugar-Free

Time: 5 minutes

1 tablespoon white sesame seeds

1 tablespoon black sesame seeds

1½ teaspoons flaky sea salt, such as Maldon

1 teaspoon poppy seeds

1 teaspoon dehydrated garlic flakes

1 teaspoon dehydrated onion flakes

This copycat spice blend comes more out of necessity than anything else. The one it mimics is not expensive and is actually pretty great! The only thing is, it's not yet available in Canada. So until everyone's favorite grocery store (rhymes with "Raider Toes") sets up shop north of the border, I'll have to settle for making my own Bagel Be Gone Seasoning. Just like with my Montreal Steak Spice (page 258), I tone down the salt content here compared to the original. If you find that it's not salty enough for your taste, simply increase the salt in increments of ¼ teaspoon until the flavor of the blend works for you. Note that using a finer-grained salt, such as kosher salt, Himalayan pink salt, or fine sea salt will make this saltier because of more salt per given volume than the larger flaky sea salt crystals. (In other words, a teaspoon of Diamond Crystal kosher salt is saltier than a teaspoon of Maldon flaky sea salt.)

In a small jar, combine all the ingredients. Seal the jar and shake to combine. Store in a cool, dry place for up to 1 month.

JERK RUB

An intensely flavored and spicy rub that is as versatile as it is delicious. Use it to make my Jerk Chicken (page 55), Jerk Ribs (page 142), or grilled fish such as red snapper. Make sure to wear gloves when removing the seeds from the Scotch bonnet chiles—they are super spicy, and the last thing you want to do is accidentally get some in your eyes!

    For best results, let the rub sit on whatever you're marinating for at least 4 hours so the flavors have time to develop and penetrate. Any leftover rub can be stored in the refrigerator for up to 5 days or in the freezer for up to 6 months.

In a food processor or blender, combine all the ingredients and blend on medium speed until smooth. (Alternatively, combine all the ingredients in a widemouthed mason jar and blend with an immersion blender until smooth.) Transfer to a jar, cover, and store in the refrigerator for up to 1 week.

6 scallions, white and light green parts only, coarsely chopped

¼ cup coconut aminos

2 Scotch bonnet chiles, seeded

2 tablespoons apple cider vinegar

2 tablespoons avocado oil

3 garlic cloves, coarsely chopped

1 tablespoon grated fresh ginger

1 tablespoon fresh thyme leaves

1 tablespoon whole allspice berries

1 teaspoon freshly grated nutmeg

Gluten-Free

Dairy-Free

Whole30

Paleo

Grain-Free

Sugar-Free

Time: 5 minutes

Note: Use a rasp-style grater, such as a Microplane, to grate the nutmeg.

SAUCES, DRESSINGS, AND SPICE BLENDS

MONTREAL STEAK SPICE

Gluten-Free
Dairy-Free
Whole30
Keto-Friendly
Paleo
Grain-Free
Sugar-Free

Time: 5 minutes

2 teaspoons coarse sea salt

2 teaspoons dehydrated onion flakes

2 teaspoons dehydrated garlic flakes

2 teaspoons red pepper flakes

1 teaspoon dill seeds

½ teaspoon coarsely ground black pepper

Montreal steak spice is undoubtedly my mother's favorite thing in the entire world. Growing up, she would put it on absolutely every-thing, not least of which is her famous roast chicken (see page 69). She still uses it to this day, so I decided to make it from scratch to tone down the sodium level a bit. It works wonders on grilled vegetables, chicken, beef, or lamb!

The measurements given here make enough seasoning for 2½ to 3 pounds of meat. Feel free to make a larger batch; just keep the proportions the same.

In a small jar, combine all the ingredients. Seal the jar and shake to combine. Store in a cool, dry place for up to 1 month.

UNCLE RONNY'S MAGIC DUST

Gluten-Free
Dairy-Free
Paleo
Grain-Free

Time: 5 minutes

2 tablespoons coconut sugar

1 tablespoon granulated onion

1 tablespoon granulated garlic

1 tablespoon sweet paprika

2 teaspoons kosher salt

1 teaspoon cayenne pepper

This is my go-to spice rub for all things BBQ and grilling. It's absolutely perfect for smoked or grilled chicken and ribs! The coconut sugar is not Whole30-compliant, but it is Paleo-friendly. It adds a subtle sweetness, caramelizes beautifully on the grill, and balances the spice from the cayenne.

In a small jar, combine all the ingredients. Seal the jar and shake to combine. Store in a cool, dry place for up to 1 month.

RAGIN' CAJUN SPICE RUB

If you're looking for an all-purpose blackening spice, this is it! Feel free to make it as "ragin'" as you like by adjusting the cayenne pepper to taste. You're the boss, applesauce! Use it to make my Ragin' Cajun Wings (page 51) and Cajun Cod with Red Pepper and Spinach Cream Sauce (page 177).

In a small jar, combine all the ingredients. Seal the jar and shake to combine. Store in a cool, dry place for up to 1 month.

1 teaspoon granulated garlic

1 teaspoon sweet paprika

1 teaspoon kosher salt

½ teaspoon freshly ground black pepper

½ teaspoon smoked paprika

½ teaspoon dried oregano or thyme

½ to 1 teaspoon cayenne pepper (use the higher quantity if you like more heat)

Gluten-Free

Dairy-Free

Whole30

Keto-Friendly

Paleo

Grain-Free

Sugar-Free

Time: 5 minutes

SHAWARMA SPICE

Gluten-Free
Dairy-Free
Whole30
Keto-Friendly
Paleo
Grain-Free
Sugar-Free

Time: 5 minutes

1 teaspoon granulated onion

1 teaspoon ground cumin

1 teaspoon ground coriander

1 teaspoon kosher salt

½ teaspoon ground turmeric

½ teaspoon cayenne pepper

½ teaspoon ground cinnamon

½ teaspoon ground cardamom

It took me a year of playing around with different ratios and combinations before settling on this shawarma spice blend, and I couldn't be happier with the result. Use it to make my Chicken Shawarma (page 52) and be sure to try it on roast or grilled lamb!

The measurements given here make enough seasoning for about 2 pounds of boneless, skinless chicken thighs. For larger batches, increase the quantities but maintain the proportions.

In a small jar, combine all the ingredients. Seal the jar and shake to combine. Store in a cool, dry place for up to 1 month.

TACO SEASONING

Skip the store-bought stuff and throw together this taco seasoning in a matter of minutes using a handful of readily available spices. Use it while sautéing ground beef, chicken, lamb, or even shrimp.

The measurements given here make enough seasoning for 2 to 2½ pounds of ground beef. For larger batches, increase the quantities but maintain the proportions.

In a small jar, combine all the ingredients. Seal the jar and shake to combine. Store in a cool, dry place for up to 1 month.

1 tablespoon granulated onion

1 teaspoon sweet paprika

1 teaspoon ground coriander

1 teaspoon chili powder or dried ground chile of your choice, such as ancho

1 teaspoon dried oregano, preferably Mexican

1 teaspoon ground cumin

¾ teaspoon kosher salt

½ to 1 teaspoon cayenne pepper (use the higher quantity if you like more heat)

¼ teaspoon freshly ground black pepper

Gluten-Free

Dairy-Free

Whole30

Keto-Friendly

Paleo

Grain-Free

Sugar-Free

Time: 5 minutes

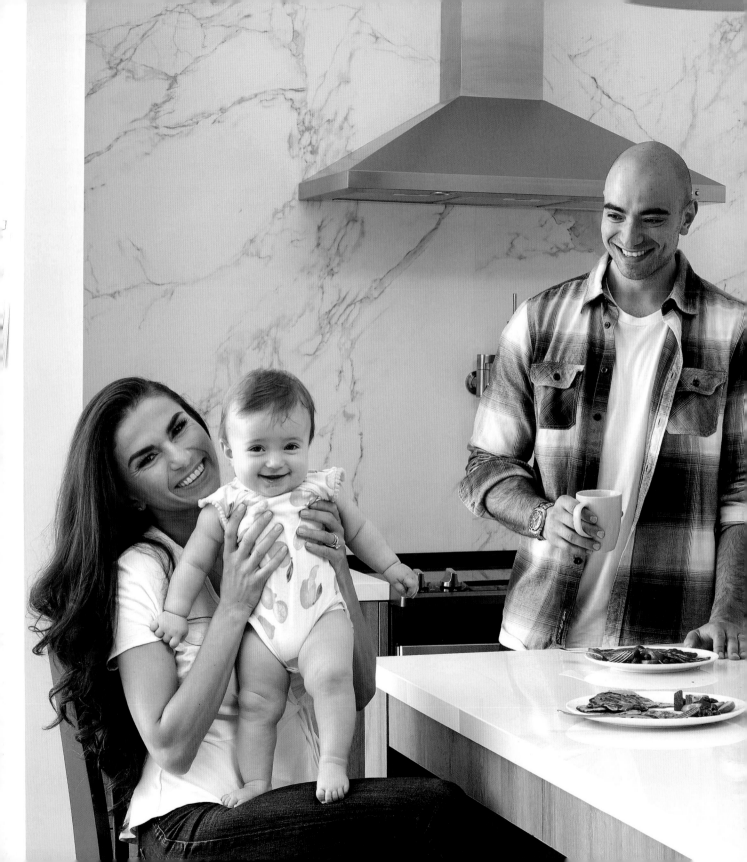

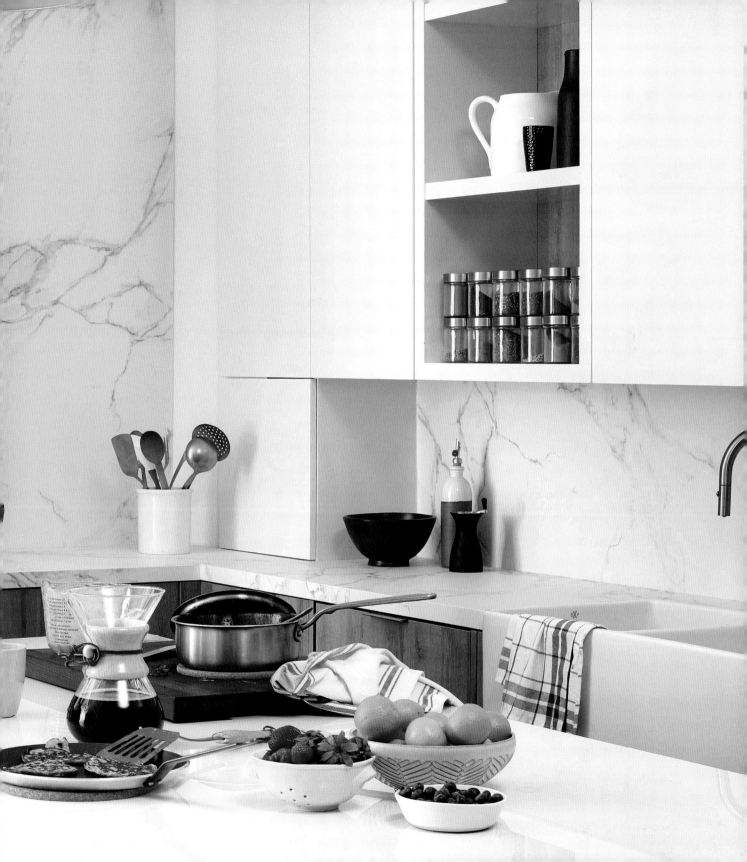

INDEX